Attitudes
of Play

Attitudes of Play

Gabor Csepregi

McGill-Queen's University Press

Montreal & Kingston • London • Chicago

© McGill-Queen's University Press 2022

ISBN 978-0-2280-1407-2 (cloth)
ISBN 978-0-2280-1408-9 (paper)
ISBN 978-0-2280-1502-4 (ePDF)
ISBN 978-0-2280-1503-1 (ePUB)

Legal deposit fourth quarter 2022
Bibliothèque nationale du Québec

This book has been published with the help of a grant from the Federation
for the Humanities and Social Sciences, through the Awards to Scholarly
Publications Program, using funds provided by the Social Sciences and
Humanities Research Council of Canada.

Printed in Canada on acid-free paper that is 100% ancient forest free
(100% post-consumer recycled), processed chlorine free

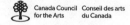

We acknowledge the support of the Canada Council for the Arts.
Nous remercions le Conseil des arts du Canada de son soutien.

Library and Archives Canada Cataloguing in Publication

Title: Attitudes of play / Gabor Csepregi.
Names: Csepregi, Gabor, author.
Description: Includes bibliographical references and index.
Identifiers: Canadiana (print) 20220273308 | Canadiana (ebook) 20220273324 |
    ISBN 9780228014072 (cloth) | ISBN 9780228014089 (paper) | ISBN 9780228015024
    (ePDF) | ISBN 9780228015031 (ePUB)
Subjects: LCSH: Attitude (Psychology) | LCSH: Play.
Classification: LCC BF327 .C74 2022 | DDC 152.4—dc23

To Thomas De Koninck,
a steadfast guide and a dear friend ever

Contents

Acknowledgments

I wish to express my profound gratitude to Professor Paul D. Morris for carefully reviewing the manuscript and making precious recommendations for its improvement. I also extend my sincere thanks to Khadija Coxon at McGill-Queen's University Press for her generous and practical counsel. And I am most grateful to my wife, Éva Balázs, for her continuous encouragement and playful inspiration.

Attitudes
of Play

Prologue

For some time I have been thinking about the presence of playful elements in human behaviour that, at first glance, have little to do with play itself as we perform or observe it. We take our early morning stroll across a park and whistle a tune. We bring a touch of humour into greeting a neighbour or taking part in a community soccer game. We notice lovers or business associates freely bantering back and forth, making their interaction lighthearted and pleasurable. Yet we seldom refer to these activities as play or assign them the term "playful." Perhaps we need C.S. Lewis's reminder that "Venus is a partly comic spirit" and "makes game of us."[1] Hermes too, the patron of merchants and traders, liked to disguise himself and play practical jokes on both gods and humans.

If we approach the domains of Venus and Hermes with deferential gravity rather than carefree humour, it is undoubtedly because we are disposed to consider play as an activity that is distinct, separate from what amorous persons or business partners occasionally enjoy. The widely read analyses and reflections of Johan Huizinga (*Homo Ludens*) and Roger Caillois (*Man, Play, and Games*) confirm such views; these authors have regarded play as unmistakably distinct from other sorts of human doings. Still, they have not failed to notice that there are activities in our day-to-day existence that can hardly be called play but are nonetheless accomplished in the *spirit* of play – with an *attitude* of play.

In the present volume, I undertake a cursory analysis of play. *Yet I do not propose here another book on play.* The object of my enquiry is the play attitude, which, as I shall suggest, grows out of play and is usually adopted while playing, but which, even so, is distinct from play and embraces a much wider scope. I want to show that this attitude can be the mainspring or accompaniment not only of play itself but of all sorts of human activity and behaviour. I therefore view play both as an activity and, in the words of Émile Benveniste, as a "certain *modality* of all human activities."[2] I consider this *modality* a certain *ethos*, disposition, outlook, or thought with which an activity is carried out, whether within or outside the sphere of actual play. The reflections in this book are about human ways of being playful and acting playfully in the world. My intent is to delve into the persisting human tendency to take up – spontaneously or deliberately – a play attitude toward any kind of human experience. While many excellent books and articles have been published on the importance of play in human cultures and, more recently, on the beneficial functions of play activities in educational contexts, too little attention has been paid to the central role of play as an attitude toward human life.

This study is intended to be extensive but not exhaustive. Beyond what I consider important to highlight, further characteristics and concrete appearances – common and uncommon – of the attitude of play may be revealed and analyzed. I hope, therefore, that my outline is convincing enough to induce readers to turn to their own experiences, look for examples in their own lives, and complete and deepen what is said here.

Although an attitude of play can be practised and observed in its manifestations and contexts in almost every department of our lives, it defies analysis as an exclusive entity because it cannot be detached and isolated from concrete activity and seen in pure form. We may perceive its action, but the attitude that shapes it manifests itself only in part or escapes our notice altogether. Indeed, an attitude of play can manifest anywhere. For this reason, in the following pages, I turn my attention mainly to everyday occurrences and to experiences shared by people of diverse ages, backgrounds, and cultures.

Creative achievements in science and art have often been linked to play, and it is not uncommon to detect an attitude of play in the works of outstanding jesting figures of the past such as Rabelais, Erasmus, or Joseph Haydn.[3] A playful attitude can also be an important aspect of present-day ordinary human life, manifesting in a great variety of circumstances not only in childhood but through all stages of becoming. If I mention outstanding historical personalities, it is because I see them as models that all of us may emulate in our individual contexts. As we shall see, we may grow into an attitude displayed by a person we hold in esteem and gradually make it our own.

My interest in this detailed study of play attitude was sparked by observing people's activities in the workplace and in leisure settings. I noticed that people who approach their daily tasks or recreational pursuits with an attitude of play seem to lead a happier and fuller life. They may experience disappointments, become embroiled in conflicts, meet with failures, or, as we shall see, occasionally lose touch with reliable guidance for their conduct. Nevertheless, no matter how strong the headwinds they may face, they maintain a cheerful and good-humoured stance to life, hold fast to their own playful disposition, and find in it and its underlying qualities ways of learning and practising the art of life. The celebrated inventor Ernő Rubik, in his recent book *Cubed*, has voiced an opinion that goes to the heart of the matter: "Too often as adults we seem to believe play is just a diversion, or another form of competition outside of the workplace. But play is one of the most serious things in the world. We often do things really well *only* when we do them playfully. We are more relaxed about them; the task becomes not a burden or a test, but an opportunity for free expression."[4] On reading this, I asked myself: what kind of attitude allows people to do things playfully, to be more relaxed and to carry out their tasks with ease, subtlety, and expressive freedom?

In certain quarters of public life, by comparison, I have also noticed, not without a certain astonishment, people's inability to accept an attitude of play in interactions with colleagues, representatives of institutions, fellow travellers, even friends – in short, all those they happen to meet in the hustle and bustle of their daily lives. It seems that their everyday worries and trepidations or an overarching despondency colours their words and actions, and makes them immune to the spirit of unguarded playfulness. I have also noticed a complete humourlessness and unctuousness in exchanges in some professional circles. The corresponding absence of qualities pertaining to human interaction – tolerance, acceptance of flaws, and regard for the whole truth, for instance – has reminded me of the oppressive atmosphere created by totalitarian political systems. The ability to listen to people who see the world in a different way, and the capacity to admit that they might be right after all were non-existent in these milieus of exaggerated rigidity. In such settings I observed that humorous comments, teasings, and pranks were banished from certain dried-up public institutions; people were inclined to adopt a cautious, remote, and unsmiling manner, guarding their tongues or filling their conversations with a set of stock responses. Such situations bring to mind Heinrich Rombach's admonition to initiate and maintain human communication or to accomplish professional assistance with genuine humour: "Hardly anything is more important for humans than humour and it is very sad that this unparalleled educational objective (*unüberbietbare Bildungsziel*) appears nowhere in our educational plans."[5]

I have been able to confirm the relevance of observations by influential philosophers on the rise of abstractness in our societies today, the loss of the immediacy of sensory experiences. These scholars have pointed out that a progressive severance of words and of gestures from the solidity of tangible realities is a key symptom of our age. Because of the widespread tendency to use technological devices and machines in our private and public environments, active sensory engagement with our material environment is becoming increasingly rare. In our communications, we prefer abstract symbols and images over bodily presence and become more and more "unworldly." We tend to use abstract notions in speaking and writing rather than words referring to concrete things. Consequently, we become blind and deaf to the language of things and, with the growing distance between ourselves and our ambient surroundings, ever more passive. We no longer believe in the aliveness of familiar objects and fail to perceive their messages, the meaning and value that they hold for us in everyday situations. We seldom live such "blessed moments" as Pascale Rouet describes, when a musical instrument, an organ or a piano for instance, flares up, gets animated, and seems to become a breathing being, an extension of the player's living and sensible body.[6]

Bodiless language, humourless professional mood and practice, disengagement from active sensory communication with animated environments, and other forms of abstract behaviour result in a disregard for aesthetic values as well as the waning of the play attitude. Aesthetically sensitive visitors to major cities bemoan a lack of creative imagination, an absence of the nourishment of *choses vues, touchées, goûtées* in recently built residential sections. Children who walk on streets lined with uniform, algebraic, and well-groomed houses are not as eager to adopt a play attitude as their comrades who live in neighbourhoods where they meet life in its untidy manifestations. Reflecting on the dull uniformity of suburban environments, Lewis Mumford has noted in *The Urban Prospect*: "Animation, though at the price of a little disorder, is more exhilarating, even esthetically, than frozen respectability."[7]

We may imagine that a derelict environment, a dismal and forbidding atmosphere, stifles the play attitude. But even under such austere conditions as prevail, for instance, in prisons or in the slums of industrial cities, some people are able to adopt an unexpectedly lighthearted approach to their fellow human beings and even to their own fate. They find the capacity to rise above their dire situations, the drab ambience of their circumstances, their apparently unchanging world, and discover or imagine a form or a behaviour that evokes in them a playful mood. They are somehow able to take on a new sense of self and transcend whatever at first seemed repulsive, desolate, and unchangeable. To refer to another observation by Lewis Mumford, even bombed-out areas of cities, with their rubble, exposed cellars, and bare façades, can serve as inviting playgrounds for the fancy of children.[8]

Another phenomenon that has caught my attention in the past ten or fifteen years is the controlled design of living spaces – such as the playgrounds in our neighbourhood – in which excessive concern for safety induces conformity and compliance rather than inventiveness and free play. Children of our time seem to have fewer opportunities to take risks and trust in a fortunate turn of events. Parents, teachers, and urban planners are more concerned with creating safe, secure, and risk-free environments than with making it possible for children to move with ease and, free of stifling rules and prohibitions, to explore all sorts of milieus and create imaginative adventures. Yet recent studies have shown that refraining from excessive protection and preventive measures and actions often brings significant gains: children learn to trust their own judgment, face uncertainty with confidence, and make far-reaching and daring decisions. In environments where they learn to consent to the risks of the world while being actively involved first in adventurous play and later in daring physical activity, children can gradually acquire emotional maturity. As they grow older, they may become involved in sports activities that bring the delight of risk into their lives. Attempts to attenuate or neutralize risk are pernicious elements of our contemporary life, and I will make a few remarks on the prevalent eschewal of uncertainty, which tends to produce situations in which the adoption of an attitude of play no longer has any relevance.[9]

Although I deplore all these social circumstances and changes, it is not my intention to analyze at length the causes of the absence of an attitude of play in our lives, exemplified by the inability to cultivate an awareness of the present and remain attentive to the "language of things," the waning of courtesy and elegance, the vanishing of spirited and disinterested conversations caused by the ubiquity of cell phones and the omnipresence of debilitating background music, or the dismissal of the superfluous and the beautiful in created objects and accomplished actions. As in my earlier book on the defining moments of human existence, I want to deal here as much as possible, as Rubik has proposed, with the positive and constructive side of human life and, celebrate those experiences that bring us fulfilment and enhance our freedom and our love of ourselves.[10]

It has become customary to emphasize the significance of play in the development of a child's future personality. Play attitudes and activities are recognized as primary means by which children learn to express feelings, control aggressive tendencies, become disciplined, cooperate and deal with loss, acquire perseverance, think their own thoughts, and establish a relation between fantasy and reality. Far from being a way of escaping from the world, diversion, as Blaise Pascal suggested centuries ago, can be seen as a way of entering into the world and developing selfhood in this world.[11] Jacques Henriot, in his book *Le jeu*, goes even further: "Play appears as the movement through which human beings make themselves human."[12] Jerome Bruner's "Play, Thought, and Language" gives a still more specific valuation of play in human life: "To play is not just child's play. Play, for the child and for the adult alike, is a way of using mind, or better yet, an attitude toward the use of mind. It is a test frame, a hot house for trying out ways of combining thought and language and fantasy."[13] Through a playful approach to realities, children learn to summon absent realities and develop a capacity for generalization even before they can use linguistic symbols. Productive thought, the habit of persistent inquiry, the capacity for the creative use of language, and the fulfillment of human relations all require agility in "the use of mind." The ability to see oneself from a distance, to imagine oneself being someone else and to become someone else, and thus define oneself as both the author and actor of one's own activity – these are all salutary outcomes of intersubjective play.[14]

While reading various valuable contributions to our understanding of play, I felt the temptation to follow suit and regard manifestations of the attitude of play, partly or entirely, as a particular means by which specific educational objectives are achieved. My focus, then, would have shifted to the ways in which a playful attitude helps one learn and grow in knowledge, imagination, and wisdom. I have tried, however, to resist this temptation to unduly emphasize the educational value of an attitude of play, in part also because to do so would risk becoming purely utilitarian, betraying the very essence and role of play. I am inclined to think that it is more important to allow students to learn how to live well than to bombard them with edifying directives and duties. I believe that play attitudes and activities can be valued not merely for their didactic benefits but also, and chiefly, for the overall fulfilment and joy they implicitly offer. I am guided by the conviction that a life without humour, risk, or attentive receptivity to animated forms would be much poorer – flavourless, and uniform; it would lack lustre and zest. The attitude of play deserves to be described, explained, and valued without giving in to the urge to praise its benefits beyond measure and insert it into an educational plan. To quote a slightly amended remark of Bruno Bettelheim: "The greatest importance of play attitude is the child's immediate enjoyment of it, which extends into an enjoyment of life."[15]

I must admit, however, that, while I was thinking of the actions and values that we need to uphold for the younger generation, a sobering warning for our times advanced by John Berger often came to mind: "The culture in which we live is perhaps the most claustrophobic that has ever existed; in the culture of globalisation, as in Bosch's hell, there is no glimpse of an *elsewhere* or an *otherwise*. The given is a prison. And faced with such reductionism, human intelligence is reduced to greed."[16] I maintain that, by taking an attitude of play, we have a chance of gaining access to an "elsewhere," acting "otherwise," and guiding our mind away from hoggish self-interest and stifling uniformity. We become able to focus on the intrinsic meaning of things while at the same time exploiting or ignoring their practical utility. My reluctance to treat this kind of freedom from the perspectives of functionality and pedagogical and remedial usefulness does not mean that I do not wish to see it rooted in ethical and aesthetic values. I have been fully aware of the cautionary note of Antoine de Saint-Exupéry, who, in his *Terre des hommes*, disdained risk-taking that was not grounded in an "accepted responsibility" and saw it as a "sign of poverty and excess of youth."[17] Such considerations suggested that there was another temptation to avoid: detaching elements of the attitude of play from fundamental ethical and aesthetic concerns and replacing their comprehensive anthropological description and genuine praise with blind and narrow idolatry.

For this study, I have drawn upon lesser-known works as well as often-quoted sources, chiefly upon the contributions of F.J.J. Buytendijk. Buytendijk's emphasis on the *pathic* aspect of the reciprocal communication we have with things and people is essential for a thorough understanding of both play and play attitude. I find it therefore unfortunate that, unlike the classic works of Johan Huizinga, Roger Caillois, Eugen Fink, and Hugo Rahner, as well as the theory of play developed by Hans-Georg Gadamer in his *Truth and Method*, Buytendijk's systematic study on play has not yet been translated into English and thus remains largely unavailable to a wider audience. I agree with Helmuth Plessner, who in a note appended to his observation on play's "paradoxical relation which enables us to commit ourselves, yet without becoming so firmly established that individual choice is completely lost," declared: "Buytendijk's formulation in his *Het spel van mensch en dier als openbaring van levensdriften* (The Play of Humans and Animals as Manifestation of Life Instincts) is the best analysis of play we have."[18]

In the course of my reflections on the presence and absence of play attitude in our conventional life, a remark by Hungarian poet Attila József, made in 1936, also struck a chord in me: "I don't understand why play, the joy of children, should be seen as something inferior. During my happy moments, I feel as if I was a child. My heart is serene when I discover in my work occasions to play. *I am afraid of persons who are unable to play* and I will do what I can to keep alive people's playful mood and to stamp out all the constraints which undermine the spirit and possibility of play."[19] What kind of person is it who is unable to play, to introduce a spirit of play into an activity, and take an attitude of play? The compulsive person, fixated on the search for certainty and perfection, unable to change daily routines or improvise an action spontaneously without concern for its outcome, is a person unable to adopt a play attitude. Likewise, the fanatic person, who adheres to a given set of ideas and uses violent means to convert ideas into reality, is surely never visited by a playful mood. We find a frightening illustration of the fanaticized mind in Frank Pierson's well-known film *Conspiracy*, in which Adolf Eichmann vehemently rejects the manifestation of two forms of pure play: the uniformed chauffeurs laughingly throwing snowballs at each other, and the sublime Adagio movement of Schubert's *Quintet in C Major*. What more fitting way to warn us about evil than to portray inflexible individuals who detest redeeming experiences that arise from an instinct for play – laughter and music – experiences that elude the austere and ruthless logic of expediency and intimate an ideal image of what life could be.[20] And, similarly, how right was G.K. Chesterton with his reflection on the education of future political leaders: "I would much rather be ruled by men who know how to play than by men who do not know how to play."[21]

I have, then, asked myself: what are the human qualities in our contemporary life that could counter the pernicious influence of fanatical rigidity and compulsive pedantry, foster the spirit of play, and provide opportunities to shape our destinies freely, fearlessly, and above all, peacefully? I agree with André Leroi-Gourhan, who has offered an insight into the evolutionary origin of our humanity: "I should like to think that humour was the first invention of human being, the first condition of his survival."[22] Humans, he suggests, were able to survive because their plays and play attitude, in the form of humour or purposeless and generous acting, sought to create a common ground of understanding, collaboration, and recognition. Ferdinand Ulrich too doubtless thought about this kind of serene and tolerant coexistence when he proposed this concise definition: "Play is the guarantor of peace."[23]

The reader will find in this study a constant appeal to immediate experience. I consider concrete situations in which individuals, young and old, adopt a play attitude and, thanks to a temporary or lasting change in their inner disposition, modify for a longer or shorter time their way of relating to their fellow human beings and their environment. By turning to the lived manifestations of this altered relation – loving relationships, sport and leisure activities, conversation, leadership practices, teaching and lecturing, strolling, drinking wine – I hope to contribute to a better understanding of the attitude of play and to reflect on its existential implications. The first step in exploring this theme is to clarify the concept of attitude and to highlight its central importance. Thereafter, I would like to show that the five ways of adopting a play attitude are rooted in play, in its most complex and prevalent forms, and that they can influence or favourably guide human behaviour beyond the realm of play. And further, I want to dispel the notion that instilling humour and fun into our activities is synonymous with being frivolous and undignified; and I will offer examples of how adopting an attitude of play allows us to experience well-being and moments of genuine happiness.

1

The Concept of Attitude

n our daily existence, as we move to and fro in our personal and wider worlds, we encounter a great variety of attitudes; we see others, for instance, as friendly, gloomy, critical, contradictory, tolerant, generous, reverential, polite, collegial, indifferent, arrogant, or ambivalent. People take attitudes according to the practical social context in which they find themselves, or as they are influenced by ideas, values, and norms that they may hold deeply all their lives or only for a certain time. We see athletes taking part in competition with a winning attitude and leaders guiding their organizations with a collaborative, respectful, and broad-minded attitude. Such attitudes are formed and displayed in every domain of our everyday lives: in our professional milieu, in leisure activities at home or travels abroad, in educational institutions, in political gatherings or artistic performances, as well as in periods of illness and other sorts of misfortune. Attitudes endow our interactions with people and objects with specific qualities; an attitude may be solemn, attentive, impartial, informal, submissive, pacific, dominant, brazen, joyful, surprised, balanced, generous, philosophical, courteous, diplomatic, scientific, or playful, among many others. It may happen that an attitude blends two seemingly opposite traits: passion and impassiveness, or friendliness and aloofness.

We sometimes reflect at length and even consult friends or colleagues on the type of attitude we ought to take when we receive a job offer or when we read about a strike action proposed by employees of a transport company. There are also occasions when we display an attitude without even thinking about our reason. When we hear about a person being invited to give a lecture on a contentious topic and subsequently, after a ritual of denunciation, being pushed out of public debate, our internalized values and norms, as well as our moral makeup, instantaneously generate either approval or disapproval of the decision.

Students of social psychology may see an attitude as providing an evaluative viewpoint and disposition for the acting persons in their orientation toward the world. When we deliberately take an attitude, we evaluate both the situation in which we find ourselves and the appropriate mode of action that, for others and ourselves, suits the situation. When we have to communicate an unpleasant decision to someone, our words, tone of voice, and bodily posture express a tactful attitude. As we enter a store or a public office, we immediately perceive attitudes – expected or unexpected – that may influence our own attitude. Perceived attitudes tell us what sort of behaviour is appropriate or inappropriate and what kind of communication on our part will elicit approval or disapproval. "The term 'attitude,'" in the words of Charles Leslie Stevenson, "designates any psychological disposition of being *for* or *against* something."[1]

From the perspective of philosophical anthropology, an attitude is a way of relating to someone or something in our life world.[2] An attitude establishes a relationship with persons and things, and endows the relationship with distinct characteristics, which in turn generate thoughts, feelings, actions, and judgments. An attitude shows preference for a particular approach to an activity, a profession, an institution, or a community. In some instances – as when one applies for a professional work position – the desired approach toward objectives and tasks is sometimes deemed even more important than previously acquired knowledge, experience, and skill. An attitude of openness and friendliness toward outsiders may lead to their concrete acceptance within a well-knit community. An attitude of curiosity toward a scientific path may prompt someone to study, make experiments, advance hypotheses, observe, and eventually initiate a planned research activity in collaboration with others. A phenomenological attitude on the part of a philosopher leads to an intuitive and receptive experience of things – what Max Scheler describes as "the most vital and most immediate contact with the world itself" – and, as such, precedes discussion of whether an experienced thing is true or false, genuine or worthless, authentic or inauthentic, real or illusory.[3] Upon reading a philosophical work, one might conclude that the author adopts, with regard to human condition, either a cosmocentric or an anthropocentric attitude.

Otto Friedrich Bollnow posits the voluntary nature of attitude: an attitude (*Haltung*), he says, "is a freely chosen state of mind (*seelische Verfassung*) that one has 'taken' on his own."[4] Feelings and ideas may come to us without our consent; attitudes we choose of our own accord. For this reason, we are responsible for the attitudes we adopt whether swiftly or after lengthy reflection. We assume and display an attitude toward something we consider significant and relevant in our lives: learning a language, making money, teaching young ones, or preserving an ecological balance. We may at times consider the seemingly insignificant to be worthy of our attention and thereby make it significant. Endowing something with significance is a prerequisite to the adoption of an attitude toward it, even if we relate to it with aloofness or reserve, or submit it to an objective and impartial observation. Just as there are in everyday affairs any number of realities to which we accord significance, there are any number of approaches that we may take toward these realities: we may observe, study, discover, question, analyze, use, develop, transform, imitate, admire, and enjoy them. (The adjectival form of each of these verbs indicates the form of attitude that we may assume while we relate to things and people.)

In a text entitled *What Is Enlightenment?*, Michel Foucault proposed a comprehensive definition of attitude. "By attitude I mean a mode of relationship with regard to actuality; a voluntary choice made by certain people; in the end, a way of thinking and feeling; a way, too, of acting and behaving that, at one and the same time, marks a relation of belonging and presents itself as a task. A bit, no doubt, as what the Greeks called an *ethos*."[5] By referring to the Greek word *ethos*, Foucault emphasized the enduring aspect of attitude. An attitude, he suggests, defines someone's personality, a habitual way of seeing the world and doing all sorts of things in this world. *Ethos* is the habit that initiates and steers our acting and is, in turn, strengthened, refined, or modified through diverse forms of acting.

The mention of habit evokes the concept of habitat, which, once again, refers to a concrete, fundamental, and durable reality; habitat is the place of residence to which we belong, where we feel at home and forge lasting and loving relationships – with a spouse, children, and friends, and with cherished objects and projects. A habitat also suggests tasks and duties of preservation, of care and embellishment. In a wider sense, habitat is the place we carry in our heart from childhood, and form and transform in our imagination; it is an inner place where the ideals of our youth continue to inspire us and the models of our present existence, with their values and qualities, provide us guidance.[6] As children, we create and treasure this place through play. Ferdinand Ulrich stressed the role of play in this early constitution and development of *ethos*: "While playing, the child takes up his domicile in the world. He places himself in an *ethos* (its original meaning is 'stable,' 'domicile,' 'habitat')."[7] This *ethos* later becomes a source of playful spontaneity, of balancing movement with rest, and of the emotional security that enables us to risk new ways of thinking and acting, and to withstand adversity and the pressure to conform to social convention.

Bollnow and Foucault passed over certain attitudes that are not adopted by voluntary choice. There are situations in which we unexpectedly and swiftly manifest an attitude without the intervention of our will. Such instantaneous responses to certain hurtful words or gestures often bring out the best in us. This is what happens when, for instance, a decision to forgive injury and forgo invective or vengeance takes place with no calculation of its beneficial or harmful consequences.

In our encounters with those who live and act around us, it is their bodily attitude that we first come across.[8] We feel welcomed when someone greets us with a warm handshake. We refer to the attitude adopted by the living body, when, for example, we praise the concrete manifestation of an idea or of a feeling with these words: "in your thought as well as in your attitude you showed …" We applaud the attitude of help and solace which visibly expresses a cherished value or ideal. While standing upright, our body may adopt a stiff, relaxed, firm, comfortable, or balanced attitude. A conversation, a visit to a museum, a participation in a religious ceremony, or the rest taken during a strenuous excursion will affect our way of standing upright. We take up a symmetrical bodily attitude in certain situations and an asymmetrical one in other contexts, and by doing so, we express respect, reverence, availability, reserve, nonchalance, openness, joy, or sadness.

An upright bodily form can express the strength of an attitude – an intention, a sudden emotion, a desire, a conviction, a thought, or a moral valuation. Or it can be a response to the seriousness of a situation; we stand up to greet someone, to show respect, to exchange vows, to manifest indignation, to contemplate a painting or scenery. Our posture when we stand in line to buy groceries differs from the stance of a worker taking a rest break, that of a security guard in front of a gate or of a toddler rejoicing in a new achievement. If we ask for a direction in a foreign city, the bodily posture of the addressee reveals immediately an eagerness to help or a lukewarm indifference. Context provides us with a clearer understanding of the meaning of bodily attitude.

Thanks to our remarkable mobility and sensitivity, our bodies are able to take positions that express other attitudes as well – bowing, prostrating, kneeling, sitting, or lying down – leading to an inflection of our relation to the world. Each of these bodily attitudes reveals the world under a certain light and conveys striking aspects of a mode of existence. In each of our bodily attitudes, we make manifest a particular mode of being and a particular way of relating ourselves to others and things around us. We praise "upright" persons who honour their obligations, who are loyal to their friends under attack or in danger, who stand by their convictions even at the risk of losing their livelihood. There are certain virtues attached to getting up early and going out to the field to till one's land, just as there are to composing a poem or a piece of music in bed, undressed and under the covers as Milton and Rossini are said to have done.

If we seek tranquillity and value stability and comfort, we sit calmly. Our body is brought to inner recollection by sitting upright and still. Saint Thomas Aquinas, commenting on an observation by Aristotle, observed: *"Quiescendo et sedento anima fit sapiens et prudens"* (While at rest and seated, the soul becomes wise and prudent).[9] Wisdom and good judgment arise out of the willingness to sit and wait patiently. Closer to our times, Charles Péguy tells us that thinkers need to be seated in tranquility and peace in order to transform an assemblage of ideas into a manageable system, into a philosophy.[10] Owing to the temptation of laziness, they keep their efforts toward an orderly arrangement of their thoughts at a distance from the activity of their lives. The German word *Sitzfleisch* (flesh to sit on), the power to remain at one's desk, has to some minds a somewhat sinister undertone today because it still connotes an over-application of rigorous efficiency and will. Pusillanimous misers "sit" on their money, which, because it is only accumulated and never spent, is rendered worthless. Wise leaders sit back, watch, and learn, acting only when they deem the moment auspicious. Deft diplomats sit down together when trying to resolve contentious issues, negotiate acceptable solutions, and reach agreements suitable to both partners. Welcoming villagers wishing to extend warm hospitality to foreigners, invite them to sit at their table and share a meal.

These examples make clear that one's body posture – standing, sitting, bowing, reclining – suggests and implies a personal or moral position or, in the words of Jürg Zutt, an "inner attitude (*Haltung*)."[11] An inner attitude refers to an enduring disposition, a lasting stance that colours one's view of the realities of a living milieu, be they stable or changing. Formed by one's ideas, values, experiences, desires, representations, and expectations, an inner attitude is what determines one's behaviour in any given situation.

Immediately observable attitudes may reveal certain traits of a human being; they are noticeable at a glance, in one's way of walking, greeting someone, engaging in conversation, or participating in public debate. The way one speaks, the words chosen, their articulation, the intonation, the acquired dialect, and the corresponding voluntary and involuntary movements all disclose both intention and character. When we speak to people, their bodily attitude immediately reveals to us their interest or their indifference. Abandonment of control over the body, as, for instance, in moments of wholehearted laughter or expressions of genuine sorrow, reveals directly, without any distortion, an inner disposition with regard to a perceived reality. Conversely, one may exert strict control over the body, in which case the ability to resist distraction and hold emotions and valuations inside also finds its expression in one's attitude.

To adopt an attitude is to make oneself present and manifest the quality of this presence. We feel the presence of a person as an overall atmosphere, which radiates an emotional tonality. Our first impression of a person occurs, often unconsciously and wordlessly, by virtue of an immediate experience of a distinctive and personal atmospheric quality. The way in which people relate to objects, actions, situations, and institutions appears in their bodily attitude; the attitude reveals whether the person is hostile, friendly, indifferent, helpful, pretentious, or demanding. We might sense in a glint of a smile an attitude of glimmering hesitation or mischievous suspicion. When meeting a revered teacher or an eminent public figure, we may be touched by their magnetic spiritual qualities; their commanding presence may exude authenticity, determination, or inner strength. We perceive these qualities even when their bodies appear to us weak and fragile.[12]

To be sure, we easily and accurately read the gentleness on a loving spouse's face or the nervousness displayed by the restlessness of a lecturer's hands. If such individuals happen to make a resolute effort to conceal or falsify their inner attitude, the attitude of "holding back," "dissimulating," or "being enigmatic" finds its manifestation through the body, which, in its slightly or more noticeably distorted or contrived form, still remains a mirror of the person. The mask that one wears communicates an attitude and elicits all manner of reactions, ranging from tactful respect to inappropriate curiosity.

An outward bearing not only indicates but also induces thoughts, feelings, desires, or representations. A change from vertical to horizontal or from a symmetrical to an asymmetrical bodily position has some bearing on how one feels and thinks about things and persons. When sports fans raise their arms high overhead, they amplify the excitement of a goal scored by their team. A slight lowering of the head intensifies worshippers' expression of devotion and respect. The formative influence revealed by the bodily expression of an attitude is wide-ranging. When we move from hesitation to resolution, or transition from passive indolence into daring initiative, we usually achieve this personal transformation under the influence of, or in congruence with, a change of posture. We picture an individual signalling resolution by standing up and the risk-averse character hedging a bet by sitting down or lying back calmly. Although Michelangelo's figure of Moses is in a seated position, the tense and drawn-back depiction of his legs, as if he were ready to stand up, enhances the intensity of the resolution expressed.

So it is that an inner attitude find its expression in an outward attitude and movement and these in turn reinforce an adopted inner attitude. They causally affect each other. Scheler has rightly pointed out that the regular performance of acts of worship reinforces one's disposition toward religious belief. A religious consciousness, he affirms, cannot be wholly developed independently of bodily expressions: "ritual is an essential vehicle of its growth."[13] Accomplishing refined and urbane actions, however small and insignificant they seem, is also essential for the development and nurturing of a sound moral disposition. Nicolai Hartmann, fully aware of the importance of this correlation, emphasized the cultivation of social graces – tact, simplicity, politeness, friendly welcome, considerateness – through the accomplishment of concrete actions. "Without established customs mankind sinks into form-lessness and savagery. Indeed, without them development of the inner ethos is hindered, because it is as dependent upon fixed forms, however superficial, as upon forms of law."[14] The fostering of such attitudes encourages a "considerable amount of heart-culture, fine feeling and humanity."[15] The same holds true for other kinds of attitudes; the more we carry out certain gestures, the more our inner attitude becomes stable and articulate and comes to shape our whole being. "Normally," declared Peter L. Berger, "one becomes what one plays at."[16] This process of personal appropriation rarely follows a prede-termined plan; through our involvement in an activity, we inevitably grow into a fundamental attitude and, conversely, having appropriated an attitude, we effortlessly behave in certain ways. And just as our behaviour proceeds from an attitude, so does our speech, all the verbal expressions that we use in communicating with others.

It would be erroneous to think that adopting an attitude in a social con-text is synonymous with "playing" this attitude – "faking" it, one might say. Admittedly, there are situations today in which we feel obliged to feign zeal-ous devotion or, on the contrary, outright resistance to a political or social cause. Nonetheless, in our daily lives, at home or at work, we are also able to spontaneously adopt a great variety of attitudes that arise from our own authentic inner makeup – we are polite, distant, spontaneous, disciplined, restless, compassionate, or reserved. We naturally and gradually grow into these attitudes according to the roles we play in our world and according to the form our culture ascribes to these roles: that is, a range of corresponding behaviours, gestures, greetings, manners, norms, and customs – the rich and diverse elements of our secondary naturalness. By adopting the required at-titude and accomplishing the variety of actions that result from a particular role, we do not pretend to be a different person, we do not do not present a façade, and we do not resort to play-acting. We are identifying ourselves with the adopted role and merely doing what that role suggests we do. We naturally and without thinking behave in a certain way and this "secondary natural behaviour" displays all the values and norms that are, in our own minds, indispensable elements of the needed attitude.[17] If we are diplomats, we negotiate as diplomats negotiate; if we are athletic coaches, we give direc-tives as athletic coaches do; if we are ticket controllers, we check the ticket of each passenger according to certain prescribed instructions. Having a model in mind, we do what is required from us to exercise properly a specific skill, trade, or function. Iris Murdoch caught this central mark of human life in her often-quoted phrase: "Man is a creature who makes pictures of himself, and then comes to resemble the picture."[18]

In a fine essay, Simon Leys, stressing the validity of this assertion, gave the example of the hero of Indro Montanelli's novel and Roberto Rosselini's subsequent film *General Della Rovere*.[19] The protagonist, initially a small-time crook, is arrested by the Gestapo and forced to enter prison as General del-la Rovere in order to obtain information from political prisoners. As time goes by, he refuses to fake the assigned role and succeeds in adopting the attitude of the army leader so effortlessly and so convincingly that, by the end, he fully identifies himself with the character and dies as General Della Rovere. When one *plays* the role of a general out of sheer obligation or fear, one merely *pretends* to be just such a national figure. But when, being truly seized by the quality of the model, one *adopts* the attitude of a general and *acts* according to the requirements of this attitude, one *becomes* a military leader, naturally and assuredly, of one's own accord.

Once an inner attitude is actively adopted and strengthened, it becomes the regulating guide for the execution of our actions. These do not necessitate a specific representation or command; we do not have to evoke deliberately a specific way of greeting in order to display the inner disposition of, for example, elegance or tenderness. Our graceful and affable way of giving a gift to a person springs effortlessly from an already formed inner attitude. If, therefore, we decide to take an attitude that conforms to our values, ideas, intentions, representations, and experiences, the corresponding movements will arise spontaneously and even with noticeable autonomy from the body.

Artistic, scientific, literary, philosophical, religious, and educational institutions and associations define and promote certain kinds of attitude for their members. We may rightly speak of the attitude of a community or a social attitude, which is in essence the collective replication of individual attitudes. Teachers wish their students to collectively emulate their attitude toward a field of study; musician conductors every now and then fear that their demanding approach to music-making will meet with a hostile attitude on the part of a whole orchestra. The term "attitude" is sometimes expressed by concepts of moral outlook, state of mind, mental makeup, style, or disposition. They all refer to the salient attitudes of people made of common clay, expressing accepted or debatable generalizations that foreign observers or local citizens eagerly magnify and emphasize. Luigi Barzini, referring to the Italian predilection for concrete objects and evident facts, has quoted this opinion of John Addington Symonds: "Realism, preferring the tangible and concrete to the visionary and abstract, the defined to the indefinite, the sensuous to the ideal, determines the character of their genius in all its manifestations."[20] National attitudes are produced, preserved, or modified over time in relation to a wide variety of realities: religions, political parties, crime, press, tradition, arts, transportation, alcohol, food, jobs, schools, sports, as well as the cultural and economic patterns and moral and political principles of social life. Attentive readers discover and identify national attitudes in literary masterpieces; others find them in a more persuasive form in humorous stories or books. The tendency to transform the fantastic into the real and, conversely, the propensity to make the real appear fantastic are revealed in humour. Humour subtly presents the instinctive fondness or aversions of national communities and their reactions to the pleasant or disturbing events of their everyday life. In this sense, Caillois has observed that the consistent and universal characteristics that regulate play and allow its classification as such exert a marked influence even beyond the domain of play; they appear at regular or sporadic intervals as the mainsprings of the human activities that men and women accomplish in all spheres of their social existence.[21]

We may take up an attitude after serious and lengthy thought and maintain it over a long period or adopt it instantaneously in response to an unexpected occurrence. Attitudes such as those involved in caring for living beings or loving family members or friends, or believing in a transcendental Being are deeply rooted in us and stem from our innermost core. Other attitudes do not have such deep roots and we may give them up gradually – or even suddenly. There are also attitudes at play in fleeting or transient moments, such as the attitude of the person who sees a work-related difficulty as if from above, with a sense of humour, or who feels at home swimming in a lake or going down a ski slope playfully and with utmost ease.

Not for all, but for many, attitudes toward forms of habitation, food consumption, clothing, travel, leisure, and entertainment present with less durability than those adopted toward a profession, a philosophical view or religious faith, or certain moral values. Circumstances of time and place exert a strong influence on people's readiness to take up or relinquish an attitude. We may think of the prevalent general human attitude to the natural environment and all the heartening or disturbing political decisions entailed.

Trends in ecological and urban thought have undergone deep changes over recent decades. Attitudes toward smoking or alcohol consumption are very different than they were sixty years ago. Modified ways of looking at exercise, nutrition, and sleep habits have a substantial impact on our health and life expectancy. Children benefit or suffer from the current shift in attitudes that parents may have adopted toward school performance or leisure pursuits enjoyed inside or outside a home. Attitudes undergo transformation and adjustment as we move from one social fabric to another, from one historical period to another. A change in attitude may occur abruptly or gradually over a longer period. In the case of a gradual development, an attitude may become stronger or weaker, more nuanced, more flexible, more attentive to the complexity of its object in its proper environment.

There are attitudes that colour our approach not only to the practical aspects of our daily life but to our whole existence and the things that matter the most to us. We may, for instance, uphold an overarching attitude related to a vocation, to what we view as the conditions and chief values, principles, and ideals of our self-realization, to what constitutes happiness and fulfilment, to what helps us to face and accept solitude, illness, and death with equanimity. The foundational attitudes upon which we build our lives involve our whole being: our reason, will, feelings, hopes, beliefs, and the memory of the decisive moments of our lives.

How do our attitudes – fundamental as well as transient – come into being? Notwithstanding individual differences, it would seem that there are a few widely shared paths leading to the constitution of attitudes. I suggest that, beyond the strong influence of the culture of a specific milieu, we acquire and develop an inner disposition toward the fundamental aspects of our lives in the same way that we acquire our own high moral principles and guiding values – from our encounters since childhood with a string of consequential persons – parents, relatives, teachers, athletic coaches, and friends. It is they who give values and principles a concrete and persuasive force and invite us to live according to them and express them in our behaviour. We recognize and welcome this force because of an inner standard of values that we already have and consciously or unconsciously apply. When we are in contact with athletes who train hard, compete with fairness, and radiate confidence and a healthy desire to win, we will most likely "catch" their winning attitude. An Olympic champion has called it a benign disease that one easily contracts. Since we cleave to such formative persons, we come to take on some of their values and form our own fundamental attitudes in harmony with them.

A similar sort of integration may occur following pivotal experiences. Witnessing outstanding achievements, social and political upheavals, or even ordinary acts of kindness and generosity exerts a strong impression on us, has a strong influence on our outlook, and defines elements of our lasting fundamental attitudes. Eminent philosophers mention in interviews and publications how their intellectual attitudes arose in response to certain events and to theoretical positions defended by thinkers in the past or present. Experiencing hardship or a prolonged illness, in one's childhood or in times of war, also has a singular formative influence. In George Orwell's case, sharing the living conditions of working-class people and observing how grinding poverty and social injustice crush their soul and body was also an attitude-defining experience. Orwell was able to develop a critical and yet nuanced attitude toward human affliction and exploitation thanks to an assignment he received by chance and the way he dealt with that fortuitous task.[22]

A virtue becomes a fundamental attitude when we recurrently manifest it in our behaviour toward others. It becomes a habit or *ethos* that prevails in all our interpersonal actions and in all situations. A commitment may become an unwavering disposition in our lives, notwithstanding any temptation to betray someone in order to achieve material or moral gains. Commitment implies a steadfast adherence to other virtues such as respect, courage, or honesty, which bring their support to make the resolute and fearless practice of loyalty possible.

An attitude, once firmly materialized through its repeated enactment, does not stand in isolation: patience leads to better understanding, kindness sustains a sense of service. A similar kind of relationship is formed between attitudes adopted intermittently. As we shall see later, one form of play attitude finds its expression in another form; receptivity to animated forms nurtures ease, and humour fosters a magnanimous collaboration between persons.

Attitudes define at their outset the possibilities of creating and entertaining human relations. Whether a relationship will be pleasant and friendly or distant and cold depends, at least for a certain duration, on the partners' initial disposition toward each other and their shared attitudes toward values (tradition, care, beauty, objectivity, for example) and certain aspects of their everyday lives (occupational and leisure undertakings, entertainment preferences, cultural interests, religious practices) that determine their interactions and the quality of their immediate surroundings.

Earlier in this chapter we saw that the attitude we adopt in the presence of another person is not always in harmony with an enduring disposition. Momentary experiences of success or of disappointment, of solidarity or opposition, friendliness or hostility are capable of generating unexpected reactions. One cannot anticipate that a person will be consistently amiable or vile; an unforeseen event could trigger unpredictable responses in them. A given gesture does not always indicate a fixed mindset. Upon witnessing the distress and helplessness of a fellow human being, a calculating social climber might spontaneously adopt an attitude of selfless generosity, abolishing the continuity between his or her past deeds and actual action. Whatever values he or she may have earlier cherished, an entirely unexpected attitude and ensuing demeanour may come forth in certain unique moments.

A previously experienced situation may also evoke a surprisingly unusual attitude. For no apparent reason one might react to the arrival of spring and warmer weather with discontent instead of satisfaction. Mourning relatives may decide to adopt an unexpectedly sunny attitude to the demise by relating anecdotes of amusing mischief from the departed person's private life rather than weeping silently.

As the above-mentioned examples show, an attitude cannot be separated from a person or a thing in the presence of which it constitutes a response. An attitude does not hang in the air in a state of isolation; it is always related to something else. An attitude is formed and finds its expression in the milieu in which individuals live as acting and responsive beings. It usually reveals itself in a concrete response to an event, an action, a situation.[23] This response may evoke a reaction, which, in turn, exerts an influence on a person's adopted attitude. A teacher adopts an attitude in response to what she considers to be the needs of her students. The interested gaze of the student audience, observed by the teacher, elicits a further response: it positively affects the original attitude.

It was doubtless experiences of this kind that prompted Erich Rothacker to see in a range of human attitudes a series of responses to situations which, in their dynamic modifications, exert their influence on the acting person. "Human life is a continuous pulsating sequence of standpoints adopted towards the fellow-player (Gegenspieler) that we call the world."[24] The term Gegenspieler as used here by Rothacker denotes both an opponent and a partner of play. The world that plays with us – a structured environment, in which living and lifeless realities have degrees of significance – first tells something and elicits a response and, once the response is given, displays adaptation and resilience. In the eyes of Rothacker, the "response" given in the form of an attitude also brings to the fore a "way of being" or a "lifestyle," which is then the object of continual modifications according to the experienced approval or disapproval of the fellow-player, the world.

The attitude of play that this scenario illustrates is one of the apt and modifiable responses to situations in which a person or a thing sends forth an appeal and produces a relation of reciprocity. In the following chapters, I shall proceed by successive approaches, in order to shed light on this particular kind of reciprocal relation between appeal and response, invitation and acquiescence, call and answer.

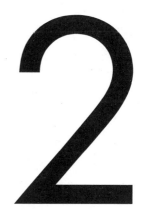

Play as Attitude

I n his oft-quoted article, the well-known French linguist Émile Benveniste speaks of the "immense domain of play."[1] What do we find in this vast domain? A great number of activities related to a great variety of tasks, rules, obstacles, circumstances, and achievements, for a start. In its widely diverse manifestations, play can also be present in our thoughts, words, feelings, decisions, movements, and deportment, in the ways of seeing an event, and in our manifold interactions with others and the world. Play appears not merely as a form of activity, but also as a way of thinking, speaking, loving someone, experiencing time and space, drawing on the resources of the body, establishing relations to living and material realities. According to Benveniste, we have a "bio-psychological inclination" to convert any regulated activity undertaken in the political, judicial, cultural, or literary spheres into play.[2] Time and again our attitude of play redefines and shapes our more serious types of occupations – teaching, healing, or worshipping – endowing them with a peculiar colouration or giving them an altogether new form and evoking in us more refined sentiments and more acute perceptions.[3] C.S. Lewis also noticed and valued this two-fold capability: "It is one of the difficult and delightful subtleties of life that we must deeply acknowledge certain things to be serious and yet retain the power and will to treat them often as lightly as a game."[4]

When we examine the experience of play on the part of the player, we can distinguish between activity and attitude. While Benveniste and a string of other past and present scholars have tended to focus their analyses on the elements and functions of play that distinguish it from other sorts of activities accomplished in our daily lives, less attention has been paid to the person who decides to play, is drawn into a play, or adopts an attitude of play. Sensitive to this neglect, Martine Mauriras-Bousquet, in her short article on the nature and function of play, has emphasized the subjective attitude associated with play rather than on the activity itself: "Play itself is an existential attitude, a way of approaching life which can be applied to everything but is not exclusively attached to anything in particular."[5]

Let us begin our analysis of this existential attitude with the following concrete observation borrowed from one of Gilbert Highet's captivating essays. Highet asserts that "play is not quite life," yet it is far from easy to see clearly the borderline between them. Given that this example also entails shifting understandings of the "rules of the game," I am not convinced that it describes a play activity, unless we look at something like a movement on a dance floor. Highet's statement presents, in a few eloquent sentences, some of the characteristics of the play attitude that may preside over a happy and carefree encounter between a man and a woman even if their situation is fraught with potentially negative consequences.

> One of the charms of serious living is that it keeps passing over into play. How often have you seen a beautiful young wife, truly devoted to her husband and children, still enjoying a little innocent play with another man? She will tease him and allow herself to be teased; she will allow him to embrace her in a gesture which, cheek to cheek, is not a real caress but a playful imitation of a caress; she will move about the dance floor in his arms, and then, when the time for play ends, when the music ceases and the crowds disperse, she will smile and stop the game.[6]

We can observe in this fictitious scenario distinct elements in the attitude adopted by both characters: an atmosphere of ease, gaiety, and humour in words and deeds, a playful imitation of affection, the temporary suspension of vital concerns, a response to movement and music, adaptability to the circumstances, a quality of restraint, and finally, genuine respect for the other person. We notice that the experience is enjoyed for itself and not for the attainment of a useful result. It provides a momentary holiday from work-related occupations. The attitude may be transposed into another similar situation and transform, for a while at least, the characteristics of conventional human relations and activities.

There are occasions when work passes into play and a task is accomplished either for the inherent satisfaction it offers or for specific communicative purposes. The following words encapsulate the experience of many, if not all, researchers: "When I write a book, I stay in a state of play rather than in a state of scientific thinking – and this does not disturb the scientific thinking; it is a matter of temperament."[7] From the paleontologist André Leroi-Gourhan we pass to the ethologist Konrad Lorenz, who convincingly asserted that creative endeavours that occur in the human mind greatly benefit from the adoption of an attitude of play. The freedom to play, to toy with ideas, is an indispensable prerequisite for the creativity of humans doing research.[8]

We find a similar statement in Patricia Highsmith's reflections on the art of writing suspense fiction: "The developing of an idea is often not at all logical, and there is such an element of play in it. I can't call the process a serious activity, though it may involve spots of hard thinking. It is still part of a game. Writing fiction is a game, and one must be amused all the time to do it."[9] D.W. Winnicott understood psychotherapy too as a form of playing: it "has to do with two people playing together." Play manifests itself in their verbal communication, "for instance, in the choice of words, in the inflections of the voice, and indeed in the sense of humour."[10] A productive and open-ended "state of play" of that nature may be experienced in the realm of entertainment or while carrying out business activities or manual work. A carpenter and a blacksmith can equally feel a sense of ease and a genuine aesthetic pleasure when producing a beautiful chair or a well-crafted lock, and can disregard, for a while at least, the monetary benefits they may derive from their activities. They are able to carry out their tasks with a play attitude when, without losing sight of an object's functional quality, they free themselves from the obligation imposed by a rigid schedule and by the requirement of valuing ends over means, quantity over quality, and similarity over individuality.

Our play attitude, either expressed or tacit, may transform and define the characteristics of many other kinds of activity. Ludwig Reiners, in his book on German prose, emphasized the ubiquity of a play attitude: "Adopting an attitude of play (*spielerische Einstellung*) is possible in all realms of our lives. It interrupts the relation to the whole of existence and takes any of its parts as a pure object allowing someone to demonstrate his dexterity and mastery as if he were moving on a gymnastic apparatus."[11] Indeed, play attitudes penetrate both the most intense and the most casual manifestations of our lives. We can detect the presence of an attitude of play in religious ritual, in diplomatic negotiations, in teaching, in commercial transactions, in athletic competitions, or in the simple act of chatting with a neighbour. It wields its influence on the creation and development of all sorts of human relations as well as on the way in which people perceive and act upon their surroundings. They may free themselves from rigid standards and constraints, take risks, or respond with a liberated mindset to unexpected invitations. They may advance humorous remarks, accomplish spontaneously unusual gestures, and drop their habitual concerns about the most appropriate ways of fulfilling social expectations, duties, and norms.

Certain philosophical works put forth learned analyses of the concept of playfulness that include the general characteristics of a play attitude. Remy C. Kwant's study of human expression, for one, defines playfulness as an attitude present in all persons who express themselves playfully.[12] When guests enjoy food, take pleasure in the wine, and find delight in the carefree exchange of views and opinions, their eating, drinking, and conversing manifest an attitude of play. "By acting in a playful way, one expresses enjoyment of life and environment: playfulness is a 'yes' to life," Kwant affirms.[13] Playfulness also "leaves room for spontaneity"; when one performs a task in a light-hearted manner, one enjoys ample "elbow room" to take initiatives, or fashion the airs and gestures of one's comportment according to individual ideas and feelings.

Playfulness may also imply a search for order in the collective execution of an activity. Participants secure the desired order when they relate to each other with "great sensitivity" and a keen sense of adaptation. Kwant also underscored the benefits of relaxation and an absence of constraint while acting with utmost concentration and seriousness. One does not have to play in order to manifest such a satisfying and cultivated playful disposition. "There are people who hardly ever play games and who, nonetheless, exist in a very playful way. There are others who make some form of playing their profession and who, nonetheless, do not exist very playfully. The playful dimension can express itself in plays and games but fortunately also outside them."[14]

Equally, Miguel Angel Sicart, a play scholar with a background in philosophy of technology, literature, and game studies, proposed a useful analysis of the concept. "Playfulness is a way of engaging with particular contexts and objects that is similar to play but respects the purposes and goals of that object or context. Colloquially, playfulness can be associated with flirting and seduction: we can be playful during sex, or marriage, or work, though none of those are play."[15] Playfulness, says Sicart, is a human capacity to introduce elements of play into any human activity or relation outside the sphere of play itself. "Playfulness is a physical, psychological, and emotional attitude towards things, people, and situations. It is a way of engaging with the world derived from our capacity to play but lacking some of the characteristics of play."[16] Sicart has proposed a concise definition of play and playfulness that I would gladly make my own: "The main difference between play and playfulness is that play is an activity, while playfulness is an attitude."[17] The play attitude we adopt extends some of the constitutive aspects of play into other types of activity – artistic, scientific, athletic, or educational. When we see a research project or a diplomatic negotiation "through the lens of play," we transfer openly or discreetly the chief qualities of play onto a scientific or diplomatic activity.[18] The foremost benefit of playfulness is "appropriation," which is a pleasurable transformation of the meaning of a situation. The new meaning elicits creativity, disruption, or expression; it brings ambiguity, colour, and depth to an otherwise straightforward, uniform, and plain activity and its context.

Normally, when we play, we take an attitude of play and, conversely, when we take an attitude of play, we are engaged in play. But we may also engage in a card game in a casino room without a play attitude; and, conversely, with an attitude of play, we may transform a seemingly tedious action, such as our walk to the corner store, into a pleasant experience of spontaneous movements. A playground swing does not automatically induce a play attitude and a play activity. Distraction, timidity, fear, or an exclusive and limited perception prompted by a work obligation (adding sand to the soil under the swing, say) may cancel out the possibility of play. We initiate play when we become receptive and open to the attraction and "invitation" of the object of play and when we adopt a genuine attitude of play. To play, as well as to adopt a play attitude, we need to free ourselves from our usual selves, abandon our usual everyday behaviour, and establish an altered relation to the things of our surroundings.

If we take an attitude of play outside the usual sphere of play – while meeting friends in a bistro, for instance – we may become aware of the tacitly adopted attitude as an overall atmosphere that discreetly affects our unfolding conversation. We enjoy hearing stories and jokes, putting forward more serious and debatable issues, and switching leisurely from one theme to another. It is only later, when we try to explain to someone why we enjoyed the evening so much, that we may compare the effortless succession of comments, interjections, arguments, and humorous observations to a playful activity, perhaps to the act of throwing a ball back and forth. We vividly recall how pleasantly and easily we nattered away with our friends, forgot our worries, and lost awareness of the passing of time. During the coming and going of questions and responses, however, we did not explicitly notice our playful approach to the occasion.

In other circumstances, we may consciously assume a play attitude even though we risk trying too hard to appear playful, and end up becoming unnatural and stiff. We may deliberately take a play attitude when, for instance, we try to dispel a tense atmosphere or defuse an adversarial situation with humour, or when we attribute expressiveness to functional objects in our surroundings or undertake our work with a sense of spontaneous improvisation. We may knowingly cultivate this attitude as an intermittent guiding *ethos* in our everyday life by seeking the brighter side of an equivocal situation and, in general, taking and maintaining, despite hardship and adversity, an equable approach to unexpected painful experiences. And, if we are able to step beyond the difficulties and petty events of our existence, we may even succeed, with the help of a play attitude, in nurturing our willingness to risk entirely new ways of seeing, imagining, and thinking the world. I believe that a play attitude helps the true philosopher to adopt and practise what Jean-François Lyotard has held as the central element of thinking: "Being prepared to receive what thought is not prepared to think is what deserves the name of thinking."[19]

As I have already pointed out, the attitude of play manifests mostly when an encounter or an event calls for an improvised response. Just as play emerges from a situation in which a thing, a word, or a gesture addresses us with

its animated and sparkling presence, likewise a play attitude requires a reciprocal relation with something that induces us to respond to it in a playful
way. Almost any phenomenon can trigger a shift from a functional and instrumental focus to an imaginative and humorous interaction. It may be a
pastime such as observing the night sky, or a professional occupation such as
cooking, nursing, or teaching that calls for concentration, strenuous work,
and passionate engagement. It is often an unexpected or sporadic surge of
uncertainty, coincidence, ambiguity, incongruity, elfishness, intimacy, or
mystery, at home, in a workplace, on a playing field, or on a journey that
elicits, spontaneously or after a moment of reflection, an attitude of play.
The play attitude is an available transient disposition that we adopt when
concrete opportunities present themselves.

We see children playing with utmost earnestness. How diligent and careful they are when they move paper ships as they engage in a maritime battle
on the carpet or, lately, on the computer screen. In all "as if" types of plays,
children willingly submit to the rules, habits, and norms of their play for the
sake of keeping to their assigned roles. Only by following prescribed and accepted rules are they able to form their play freely. Anyone who enters a game
must adopt an attitude of play consisting of accepting and respecting the existing rules: play requires committed discipline and a sense of obligation. Alain's
aphorism stresses a central aspect of play: "He who plays has sworn."[20]

It is possible, however, to turn to play without strict commitment to the
rules. Then the attitude of play consists of not being bound by the rules
and running the risk of spoiling the game. As the philosopher and diplomat
Kurt Riezler remarked in his article on play and seriousness: "We could
speak of a playful attitude if a player were to play a play within the game
itself, whether by pursuing a goal of his own or by superimposing rules
of his own on the rules of the game – replacing the spirit of the game by
the caprices of his mood, which are at odds with the spirit of the game,
although not forbidden by its rules. For example, a bridge-player might
try to get as many kings as possible in his tricks. He could be said to play
with the play."[21] Sometimes it happens that children decide not to submit
to the rules of a game, but invent and perform new ways of behaving and
impulsively determining the meaning of things. The playful attitude may
come forth in all sorts of similar inventive and mischievous detachment
from well-ingrained habits and practices, even from an already adopted play
attitude. Two persons may adopt a play attitude by light-heartedly flirting

with each other and, when they earnestly fall in love with each other, they devise another kind of play attitude to conceal their earnestness.[22] Likewise, someone may use a jovial and humorous tone in order to disguise the gravity of a risk playfully taken.

In times of festivity, the social environment demands that both hosts and guests ignore usual norms, customs, and conventions and act according to the code of the festivities. Visitors or rebels may fail to do that and perkily stray from the code. They may be most playful in their disobedience and creation of codes of their own. Similarly, writers, musicians, and diplomats sometimes decide to approach their tasks in a playful manner and cast aside certain obligations imposed by custom, language, art, or political situation. Creative translators say the same thing differently: in placing playfulness above meaning, they may favour a playful word combination over a strictly accurate use of words. When writers put into an artistic form all their previously undeclared aspirations and all the mischievous acts of their alter ego, which is often rooted in their childhood and youth, they are inspired, above all, by their inclination to replace prevailing social conventions by standards of conduct of their own invention. We might also emulate their behaviour and, in the words of Riezler, "disregard the context of ordinary life, the meaning of things, their demands, our obligations, and put in their place meanings, demands, and obligations of our own making."[23] To be sure, it is possible to adopt a play attitude even while conforming to the rules of a reality that plays with us and invites us to play: a musical piece, a form of dance, or a communal masquerade. And we may take up another form of play attitude by modifying the rules and, by doing so, changing our ways of making music, dancing, or masquerading.

For these and other reasons, the play attitude has also evoked critical voices. In one of his first major works, *Psychologie der Weltanschauungen*, the distinguished philosopher Karl Jaspers approached the play attitude (*spielende Einstellung*) with a severe eye and treated the concept of the playful with considerable disdain.[24] He declared that those who adopt such an attitude lack a genuine interest in realities. By putting realities in an imaginary context, they may enjoy their momentary experience and value some of its formal aspects: ease, lightness, cheerfulness, effortless amusement, irresponsibility, as well as all the tension, expectation, and disappointment sometimes produced by carefree behaviour. But their activities, accomplished chiefly through bodily interactions, have, he says, no relation to, or relevance for, the whole of *Existenz*. Jaspers conceded that autonomy and a certain "moral" purity may well find their concrete expression in respect for a sporting spirit and a sense of fair play. Nevertheless, the domain in which irresponsibility and levity and detachment from reality indisputably come forth is sexuality. With the adoption of a play attitude, he says, a person reduces sexuality and its social norms to the level of eroticism. "Eroticism – seldom pure – is a classic example of showing how, first, the attitude of play is short-lived and, secondly, it becomes the factitious mask, deception, and seduction for the satisfaction of base physical desires, in short unreal."[25]

In more recent times, philosophers and social critics have also considered with disapproval the attitude of what they see as unbecoming amusement and detachment from reality. Neil Postman, much influenced by Aldous Huxley's warnings about individuals' "almost infinite appetite for distraction" and their resulting "spiritual impoverishment," has deplored the ways in which television and other forms of mass communication have transformed serious experiences – political events, religious celebrations, or school learning – into pure entertainment.[26] Television presents a self-contained world that requires no sequential, rational, or complex thinking on the part of the viewer, or any critical selection and evaluation of the discourse or the succession of images. In truth, it does not call for anything other than the simple act of perception. Endless entertainment fosters passivity and offers mind-numbing distraction. The nub of the problem, of course, is not the entertainment that television offers. The crucial point is the lifestyle that the continuous availability of entertainment promotes: it consists of falling into an attitude of detachment from the realities of life and an unceasing craving for indulgence in amusement (an attitude of which Jaspers severely disapproved) and an abandonment of serious tasks and duties under the unprecedented popularity and authority of television.

In well-researched studies Robert W. Kubey and Mihaly Csikszentmihalyi have reached a similar conclusion: there is little evidence of the harmful influence of watching television, even though the majority of the programs present banal and shallow content.[27] The harm comes from prolonged exposure to television viewing. Viewers can become addicted, inactive, and unwilling to respond to the pressing and real demands of their social environment. The television screen draws viewers' attention, pulls them away from face-to-face interactions, and causes their interpersonal relationship skills to atrophy. As the philosopher Roger Scruton perceptively noticed: "Those energies and interests that would otherwise be focused on others, in story-telling, arguing, singing together or playing games, in walking, talking, eating and acting, are consumed on the screen, in vicarious lives that involve no engagement of the viewer's own moral equipment. And that equipment therefore atrophies."[28] In addition, constant exposure to televised images deprives both children and adults of the leisure to develop the richness of their own inner world – a world of thoughts, fantasies, and daydreams.[29] Because they come to experience an inner emptiness with a sense of unease, they feel the need to fill this emptiness with the most available remedy: the television screen or the computer on which they play video games. Video games involve interactivity and give users the impression of control and immediacy and a sense of engagement. However, prolonged pursuit of this screen-based form of activity fosters escapism and passive distraction, as well as an addictive attachment to the games, because of the programs' continuous adjustment of the challenges to the improving skill of the player.

It is widely acknowledged by dancers, athletes, musicians, and manual workers that the performance of skilful movements provides a pleasure independent of the attainment of a goal; psychologists call it functioning pleasure. But the pleasure found in a well-functioning body and mind depends on more than physiological processes alone; it includes also the way individuals are experiencing themselves, their acquired skills, and their relationship to the surrounding world. Konrad Lorenz has often noted that young scientists, having learned to use a computer, sought this very same pleasure inherent in other aspects of their functioning.[30] They became as children operating their first electric toy train. Innumerable individuals react nowadays to their mobile devices the same way; they play around with them absent-mindedly under the gratifying influence of their well-functioning being. Their pleasurable action becomes an end in itself and leads to a similar attitude of distraction as other forms of entertainment.

Understandably, such findings about the craving for amusement, diversion, and functioning pleasure, which is enhanced and strengthened by the ever-growing number of computer games, make a few eminent scholars inclined to treat the attitude of play with suspicion or even outright hostility. Moreover, they may question the reasons that various individuals have for not bringing elements of a play attitude into their lives. It is true that there are prim professionals who seem overly austere, hardly ever smile, and almost never advance a humorous remark. At their place of work, they may speak and act with cautious calculation and shrewd reserve. In their eyes, a playful word or gesture might open an avenue to the closeness that they want to avoid. In their intimate interactions with their loved ones, they refrain from jokes and puns, perhaps considering them unworthy, deceitful, and shallow. Whatever one's type of human makeup and underlying disposition toward play, the way one feels about oneself may well exert some influence on one's fundamental attitude. Lack of confidence in one's own abilities may silence the willingness to take risks. Those satisfied only with the perfect tend to remain impervious to humour; they rarely let their hair down or allow themselves to enjoy a hearty laugh in merry company. They seldom see themselves in a relaxed and playful manner or laugh at their own weaknesses and imperfections.[31]

We shall see in more detail that a light-hearted disposition enables one to see things and one's own existence from a slightly detached perspective with a sense of proportion and acceptance. While enjoying laughter, spouses, colleagues, or fellow workers are able to look at themselves from a distance and view their achievements and their failures both with a critical yet sympathetic eye. To emphasize this point, it is perhaps worth quoting a remark made by poet and scholar Mark Van Doren: "Nothing in man is more serious than his sense of humor; it is the sign that he wants all the truth and sees more sides of it than it can be soberly and systematically stated; it is the sign, furthermore, that he can remember one idea while he entertains another, and that he can live with contradiction. It is the reason at any rate that we cannot take seriously one whose mind and heart have never been known to smile."[32]

Some like to address their fellow human beings with gaiety, jauntiness, and refined humour. They create around them, consciously or unconsciously, a relaxed atmosphere of joviality and, whether at work or pursuing a leisure activity, can risk innovative projects with playful ease. Others, on the other hand, go through life with a demure attitude and are ready to act with carefree abandon only from time to time. They respond to unforeseen invitations to participate in communal activity, such as dancing and singing in a group on a public square, or being a cheering spectator at a football match. They may unexpectedly take up an attitude of play in other circumstances as well, as if they eagerly expected something in return, usually a fresh way of seeing themselves and their everyday experiences.

This latent human desire to see things anew brings to the fore questions about our capacity to see our visible world. In our continuous exchanges with persons and things around us, whether they are familiar or strange, we tend to see only what validates our own ideas, beliefs, and values. We relate to visible surroundings that confirm us in our habitual existence, often planned and elaborated to the last detail. How can we become aware of another, less visible, world that is hidden under the veneer of our daily lives? How can we develop our ability to see when, because of our restlessness and constant mobility, there is too much to see and our public and private spheres are filled with visual noise? How can we bring to our defensive and selective perception a quiet, integral, discerning, and nuanced observation of more complex visible realities? This is a central question repeatedly broached by some philosophers and educators.

Aldous Huxley, for one, writing about human potentialities, saw in "nonverbal education" a beneficial counterweight to the erosion of our ability to see. He strongly recommended that children be taught to relate to their surroundings in a "state of perfect ease" or "wise passiveness," with an attitude of trustful and unconcerned surrender that allows them not to immediately insert their experience into a habitual conceptual framework. This exercise of direct and unmediated perception of concrete realities, which favours the actualization of children's natural sensibility, creative spontaneity, and image-making fantasy, nurtures a playful relation to the ambient world. In addition, encouragement toward an unconceptualized and fresh awareness allows heightened enjoyment and "completely harmless happiness." It drives out boredom by bringing out the "child's play" of fantasy. Huxley compellingly argues that boredom fuels the continuous craving for ephemeral distractions (by means of various forms of passive entertainment) and enfeebles the ability to resist misleading verbiage and empty discourses. No cogent assessment of the difference between truth and falsehood seems to reach the ears of bored individuals. In a phrase, "it is useless to preach the life of reason to people who find that life is flat, stale and unprofitable."[33]

The upcoming chapters will throw light on how an attitude of play also allows us to perceive new forms and new meanings in our everyday world. When that takes place, we become like children who see a picture, a vase, a bookshelf, or a sliver of carpet from an entirely fresh angle as they glimpse through the crack of a door from their hiding place in a closet. The play attitude gives us a ticket to enter another world – a world presenting expressive and dynamic qualities – which we usually fail to see or neglect to see. We envisage our practical goals with a new frame of mind, free of all assumptions about them. We gain this freedom not merely through subjective decision. We catch sight of a new world partly because the utilitarian objects of our everyday life – tables, utensils, pencils, lamps – reveal their animated and enticing presence and invite us to approach them differently.

Let us return to Highet's scenario of the dance floor and point out a hitherto-unmentioned aspect of a light-hearted and playful encounter between a man and a woman such as he described. Highet tells us that when the music and the dance stop, the playful interaction comes to a close; the participants keep their hearts intact, say goodbye to each other with courtesy and a gentle smile, and enter another phase of their everyday lives in which the play attitude is no longer appropriate; it has lost its relevance. Whether it lasts only a few seconds, or for a day or a week-long journey, the play attitude is adopted only within certain temporal slices of our lives. In its genuine form, it can be only temporary, never a constant and permanent disposition toward the tasks and events of our life. Even if we undertake an activity that puts our whole life at risk, the attitude presiding over this activity is only adopted intermittently. Risk, humour, and other forms of play attitude are islands scattered in the sea of our earnest activities and experiences. We may take on a play attitude while we prepare a meal, sing a song, change the intonation of our voice, design a web site, build a fence, play chess while soaking in a thermal bath, glide downhill on gleaming snow, skip pebbles on a water surface, read a book (perhaps even one written on play attitude!), visit a foreign village, or accomplish all sorts of other activities. Any activity that we undertake in a playful spirit has a commencement, a certain duration, and an end. It begins and concludes.

I would suggest, therefore, that a genuine attitude of play is always transient and, after a lapse of time, must give way to another form of attitude. Just as a play that never ends is no longer a play, so a play attitude that endlessly permeates the activities of daily life is not a true play attitude. Huizinga called a play attitude without temporal and spatial limitations *puerilism*. Those who adopt a never-endingly playful state of mind lack the sound judgment and critical assessment to recognize when and under what circumstances a playful approach to the world is appropriate and when it is not.[34] Today's waning of individual thought and divergent opinion, and the increased availability of trivial diversions, as well as "the marvellous development of technical facilities," facilitate the emergence and spread of a puerilistic attitude of this sort. Puerilism inevitably results in preference being given, in thought and action, to uniformity and repetitive monotony over diversity and variety – a preference that threatens to destroy a wholesome social life and the fostering of culture.[35]

The art historian Ernst Gombrich argued that Huizinga was concerned mainly with imposing limits on every form of play and playfulness. Huizinga, he wrote, "wanted to persuade his contemporaries to exercise restraint, to practise austerity and to seek the simple life … What attracted him in the model of the game was precisely this element of self-imposed discipline."[36] Admittedly, without such discipline and restraint a play attitude easily turns into a frivolous, irresponsible, and repetitive form of distraction. A funny story told by a teacher in a science class should be followed by a rigorous and detailed explanation of a scientific problem. Strolling down the street aimlessly, in a dream-like state, ideally makes way for the compassionate observation of neighbours' tribulations and opens one to the readiness to help. We must know that life as a whole is not a game; there are encounters and experiences and circumstances that do not admit of playfulness.

Correspondingly, we must also know when putting an interlocutor at ease with amicable humour is a more suitable way of acting than maintaining taciturn self-discipline. Whenever we judge it mindful of people and appropriate to their circumstances, gleams of playfulness can play a welcome role in our daily lives, if for no other reason than, for instance, to dispel the atmosphere of stifling seriousness that emanates from certain academic and professional citadels. To quote Gombrich once again: "In my own field, the history of art, we have become intolerably earnest. A false prestige has come to be attached to the postulation of profound meanings of ulterior motives. The idea of fun is perhaps even more unpopular among us than is the notion of beauty."[37] It is rather depressing to note that this observation, made in the early 1970s, has lost none of its relevance today. We may even add another adverb to Gombrich's statement: we have become *tragically* and intolerably earnest.[38]

Limiting the duration of playfulness does not make us dissatisfied. Although the activity has its origin in the past and will have its mark on the future, it makes us fully aware of the present. Whether we take part in a religious ceremony or a river canoe trip, we are no longer subject to the constraints usually prevailing when we execute an action purely with a view to the future. We tend to become more fully attentive to the immediate experience, perceive it in detail, and allow ourselves to fall under its spell. While we pursue an enchanting practical or non-practical activity, our present is no longer simply part of a temporal sequence that receives its significance only from future and past events. It is rich and complete in itself, and we have the impression that the present has extension and density. Stepping playfully outside the objective flow of time, we often experience the present moment as a deeply satisfying duration within our personal becoming. When we look back at such moments, we also notice that they are surrounded by clear boundaries.

And yet, we might run into some difficulties here too. When we undertake the ascent of a mountain in the spirit of play and suddenly experience a dizzying encounter with an abyss, the present no longer asserts its wide-openness. The awareness of risk and the ensuing feeling of anxiety throw us into the future. Practical jokes intended to deceive us by breaking the demands of social etiquette and producing disorientation and turmoil also take away the breadth of the present in which we usually linger and gradually leave behind. They pull the ground out from under our feet and we, in turning ahead in search of a solution (how can I get out of this?), find ourselves disconnected from the present. The jokers, of course, experience the present otherwise: they take delight in our momentary confusion, smile with an expression of dominance, and wait for a while before disclosing the truth or offering a felicitous escape from our perplexity.

Whether playfulness takes root in us and even becomes a cherished and cultivated attitude in our lives depends on our willingness to play and to make repeated and imaginative use of certain fundamental play elements – receptivity to appealing forms, effortless ease, startling risk, ingenious humour – and to introduce these into activities carried out beyond the sphere of play. We should readily transfer these play elements from within to without. The Swedish diplomat Dag Hammarskjöld put the matter succinctly: "In play, the body can learn the model for actions in real life."[39] I would suggest that we acquire and develop a play attitude through playing and, conversely, that we play or undertake all sorts of other activities by taking on an attitude of play. In other words, the performance of an activity creates and sustains the attitude and, likewise, the adopted attitude generates and determines the performance of the activity.

When we say that an attitude is formed through play, we may refer to the influence of particular elements – rules, field, form of movement and bodily posture, words and imitative verbal expressions, appearance of things with which one plays – which determine the progress of a play. A play attitude is mindful of the specific characteristics and tasks of the play. We adopt one form of play attitude when we try to tag another player and still another when we build a tower out of blocks and yet another when we adopt social roles and professions. Although the chosen play occurs in the relation to a well-defined task, the corresponding play attitude also displays one or more essential elements of all plays: receptivity to expressive forms, urge of repetition, independence from (or attenuation of) a useful purpose, relaxation, limitedness in time and space, and attraction to risk.

Just as we are able to throw light on the scientific or religious attitude by studying the foundational elements of a scientific endeavour or religious practice, we learn about the play attitude by tracing it back to its origin and examining the constitutive elements of play. It is in play that we find the play *ethos*, which generates a behaviour either inside or outside its sphere. In relation to the formation of this *ethos*, the observation of Buytendijk underlines the central role of carefree and creative playing with something that plays with us: "Thinking forms the thinker, composing poems the poet, playing the player, but this self-formation is shaped by *how* and *what* the thinker thinks, the poet composes, and the player plays."[40] In the following pages, I begin each chapter with certain immediate experiences of play. Thereafter, I intend to single out and discuss a particular human attitude that is formed under the guise of the *how* and *what* of play and makes itself manifest in diverse areas of our everyday lives.

3

Pathic Attitude

How and why do children start to play? asked Buytendijk in one of his studies on play.[1] We see children playing catch with a ball, skipping flat stones on the water, sculpting a human figure out of snow or sand, or making a paper airplane. We notice in their play, not without a secret feeling of nostalgia, the exuberant energy, the constant variety of movements, the relentless desire to explore. We admire their unconcern about reaching a definite goal and their ability to see a source of captivating play in a table, a ball, a crack, or a puddle on the pavement. We also know that if we were able to adopt a similar attitude and turn to things with a similar mindset, we as adults could also give ourselves over to these kinds of pleasurable activities.

What generates these deeply fulfilling play activities? What incites children to steer a model car with a remote control device or to run hither and thither among trees and feel "safe" when they touch the "home" tree? As we observe the unfolding movements, their characteristics and relations to things, we notice that play arises spontaneously from an encounter. Children delightedly splash water coming out of a sprinkler. It attracts them and generates an active relation of reciprocity. They approach the water, place their hand or their whole body under it and, laughing and sputtering, scamper away from it. They pursue this play as long as the cool water holds them in thrall and keeps alive an elementary structure of initiative and response, seizing and being seized, doing and allowing, moving and being-moved.

How, then, does sprinkling water or a ball, a hoop, a marble, a piece of cloth, or a trampoline "send" such an invitation to play? Children play with them because they see them as "animated" realities, appealing "images," presenting sensory and motor possibilities and communicating suggestions or demands to handle them in a certain way. Chairs acquire a new significance; they become a train, and therefore intimate new possibilities of approach and arrangement; their perceived dynamic qualities may undergo further innovative transformation as play unfolds thanks to the reciprocal interaction between the chair-train and the child. Children appear to become "magicians" who animate their objects of play; a marble or a block of wood is endowed with a life of its own, exerts a fascination, and invites them to pursue their enjoyable play. "Play is transformation," says Ernst Bloch, "though within what is safe and returns. As he wishes, play changes the child himself, his friends, all his things into strangely familiar stock, the floor of the playroom itself becomes a forest full of wild animals or a lake on which every chair is a boat."[2]

Referring to the constitution of the object of play, Buytendijk quotes the fine observation of Eugène Minkowski: "A thing may become animated in front our eyes, and glow, vibrate with new life, entirely different from all the habitually recognized particularities, thus emerging, without any palpable transition, from life itself and exhibiting, as a coat woven with hardly perceptible threads, all its poetry."[3] A plaything has to be, as it were, a "living" reality: one cannot play with something completely lacking a "life" of its own. A ball, a wheel, a spring, and a swing in the park are our favourite playthings because they are not indifferent, inert realities; they evoke an activity and as it were "respond" to our action. We perceive dynamic qualities in many other familiar objects – an eraser, a pencil, an umbrella, or a hammer, say – as long as we disregard or modify their habitual use. We are sensitive to their call and find ourselves drawn into a structure of reciprocal initiatives and adaptations, moving and being moved, acting and being acted upon. "Play," wrote Buytendijk in his study on the concept of encounter, "implies a world that is seen as an image with all its dynamic possibilities. We only play with something that, in turn, plays with us ... That with which one plays is never a thing that can be objectively determined. It is a form, which manifests and reveals itself in the encounter and offers itself in the interaction. Perceived as an image, it prompts, invites, and elicits the play."[4]

To play is always to play *with* something or someone. In all play, there must be something with which we play and which, in turn, plays with us. Our encounter with the object of play reveals a reciprocal structure: we spontaneously give ourselves to an experience in such a way that something could happen to us; we are both active and passive at the same time. An attitude of reciprocity finds its expression in the performance of a to-and-fro movement that renews itself in constant repetition. It is an attitude of give and take with something or someone else that makes us move back and forth in relation to it. First, we have to be "lured" into engagement by an animated reality; only after being "pulled into" the play does the interactional performance of back and forth movement occur.[5]

In his book on play, Buytendijk persuasively argues that an understanding of the essence of play comes via the clarification of the salient characteristic of "youthfulness" or "youthful dynamic behaviour."[6] Play arises from what we recognize as a youthful way of perceiving and acting. We are able to identify it through a direct intuition of moving forms. As we observe children and certain young animals carefully, we can detect in their play certain characteristics: a lack of orientation to a goal, an impulse toward movement, a lack of constancy and coherence, a certain shyness with respect to things, and a *pathic* attitude (*pathische Einstellung*).[7]

Above all, the last fundamental trait of youthfulness is essential to starting and pursuing a play activity. Let us discuss it and see how it enters our lives or becomes one of the prominent aspects of our attitude of play.

Pathic is an affective, sensual, and personal relation to the world. In the pathic sphere, we find ourselves in direct, intimate, receptive communication with things and people; we are touched by their forms, qualities, and meanings, and give ourselves to their influence. We may be enticed by a haunting melody or a charming face, or find ourselves repulsed by a garbage dump or some ugly graffiti on an old building. We relate to the things and people of our living milieu with attraction or revulsion. In a city, in a public building, or in a house, we feel we are welcomed guests or tolerated strangers. We seek either to initiate contact with or to avoid others. We are receptive to significant and noticeable realities; we are inclined to perceive and echo vivid or delicate gestures; we resonate to atmospheric impressions or symbolic qualities. We are personally affected in some way: we may be seized by the beauty of a landscape while the person walking beside us yawns with boredom. The words "echo" and "resonance" and "being seized by something" refer to our affective attunement to the outside world and our sensitivity to expressive realities: a graceful movement, a crying child, a bright and colourful vehicle, a wildly running river, or the smooth texture of a silk scarf.

The pathic relationship is either explicit or discreet. The abrupt siren of an ambulance alerts us and tells us to move aside. The atmosphere of a place of worship may elicit an affective response and guide our behaviour without our cognitive awareness. We perceive either a strident sound or a prevailing emotional ambience with a sense of availability, involvement, and participation. Both provoke in us a particular form of reaction, either conscious or unconscious: we look for the provenance and speed of an approaching vehicle; we enter an old chapel and, without thinking, slow down the pace of our walk. We yield to the demands of these impressions and respond with what seems almost instinctively to be the most suitable behaviour in a given situation.

The pathic is not limited to a receptivity to concrete and tangible realities. An encounter with something that is projected, yet, surprisingly, does not take place is also a pathic experience. It is part of the experience of play, of sport, of commerce, and other situations of our everyday lives. As Eugen Fink asserted in one of his lectures, "Play is not merely various acts, but, chiefly, human relation to possibilities and unreality."[8] The casino gambler envisages the possibility of hitting the jackpot and, more often than not, encounters its non-realization. Not receiving the expected promotion or recognition or visit of a dear friend endows a situation with a pathic quality no less than the fulfillment of the expectation.

A pathic attitude consists of being available and responding intuitively to a compelling presence or absence. Such an expression of basic human responsiveness is manifest in many areas of our everyday lives and in the nature of our relations to a multitude of things and events. We respond to the shrill sound of an alarm clock, the brisk smell of a cup of coffee, the quiet and unpretentious decency of a lecture hall, the freshness of the fruit on display at the grocer's, the brightness of a railway-crossing bar, the roughness of the stone surface under our feet, the hurtful silence of a colleague, the desolation of broken windows of an abandoned building, and many other qualities that we encounter in our surroundings. As we move about in our homes, at our work places, or in public locations, we display a readiness to be receptive to a variety of appeals addressed to us, and we usually respond to these appeals. Moving and being moved, taking initiatives and pursuing activities so that something could happen to us, these form a functional unity in our daily existence.

Of course, in many situations we are seized by an impression and are inclined to respond to its appeal without adopting a playful frame of mind. The sphere of pathic communication is much larger than the range of possible relations encompassed by a play attitude. A play attitude, as I have pointed out before, implies a complete or partial detachment from, or mitigation of, practical concerns and the perception of dynamic sensory qualities. By adopting a play attitude, we may introduce a modification into our early morning experience. Suppose we enjoy the present moment and turn our backs on future concerns. Instead of rushing out from our home and thinking about our pressing tasks, we start to improvise a simple melody on the sounds of the alarm clock; or, as we enter our work place, we detect an emotional significance in forms that we see or touch. Thanks to a momentary and brief suspension of our usual goal-oriented activities, we relate to auditory and visual forms with an altered attitude and discover new aspects of things. Alternatively, while remaining fully engaged in achieving our practical purposes, we seek to apprehend the aesthetic qualities of objects and their surroundings. We perceive the expressive languages of things beyond their practical functions.

Similarly, by adopting an attitude of play, we open ourselves to the magnetic suggestions of movement, the effects of colour, spatial dimensions such as height and depth, and a great variety of tactile and sonorous qualities. We resonate with all these vivid sensory impressions by introducing modifications into our daily activities or merely by giving "a sort of color and vim to the habitual occupations."[9]

A clear example of such a playful openness is our response to sound. Sounds exert a strong influence on us; they envelop us and reach our whole body. If we are open to impressions of sound, we can hardly resist the motor responses evoked by a clap of thunder or the music of a military marching band. We explicitly notice their power on us in a reverse manner, when we decide to turn down the sound while watching a horror movie or a football game on television. With a diminution or an absence of sound, figures and their actions lose their strong pathic appeal. We may even find them awkward or comic. Sounds are indispensable to maintaining a tension and keeping our eyes glued to the screen. We can understand, therefore, why sound is at the source of one of our earliest playful experiences. When infants hear their own sounds, they perceive them as successive "pressing invitations" to produce other sounds. They make the very pleasant discovery of being a cause of something and of exerting an influence on the people around them. Their earliest play objects are their own sounds and movements, allowing them to create the earliest form of distancing from their body and communicating with their parents and siblings. If, in this primary social group, the child's lalling instinct is reinforced and "conventionalized in social play-forms," it gradually becomes the source of a lifelong activity – singing. Suzanne Langer affirmed correctly that song is the "formalization of voice-play."[10]

The desire to experience sound sequences and intonation in connection with an attitude of play remains with humans throughout their lives. Public speakers and university professors, for instance, may find an unacknowledged pleasure in stressing or repeating words. Some of these words are unnecessarily inflated and long. While tasting the flavour of peculiar polysyllabic combinations, they make of their verbal expressions cherished toys. They suggest that they care more about the pleasing resonance of the sounds they produce and the intrinsic value of the words than about the content of their speeches.

In addressing a crowd with the sole purpose of arousing emotions and triggering latent responses, devious politicians tend to resort to empty and inflated rhetoric. There is a similarity between a child's desire to playfully evoke responses with the help of sounds and a blatherskite's intention to talk big and provoke an evangelical adherence to glittering slogans. There is no intent to convey facts or verifiable information. It is only the desire to spout sounds for the sake of manipulation that dictates the choice of words and the recourse to a repetitive incantatory style. By exploiting the pathic attitude of listeners, the sounds of a speech are intended to induce uncritical surrender to collectively shared emotions and carefully devised and concealed objectives.

An equivalent reciprocal process of give and take occurs in the realm of music. Playing articulate music on an instrument or singing, at any competence level, consists of producing rhythmically articulated tones that are in turn heard by a musician or singer and, owing to their compelling pathic appeal, elicit other tones. The tones have an impact on the musician, communicate an "impulse value," a compelling "affective appeal" to produce other tones. It is the binding, pathic aspect of tones that affects musicians and compels them to respond in some way. The tones present a range of dynamic possibilities and these, together with the score and the musician's intellectual understanding of the piece, provide the incentive to create an orderly musical continuity with relative freedom and inventiveness.[11]

If, during a leisurely stroll in a pleasant and sunny park, we happen to see a ball rolling on the ground toward us, we most likely stop, happily catch it and lob it back to those who are playing with it.[12] If we are receptive to the "pathic invitation" of the ball, we enjoy some form of contact with this simple and perfect sphere. Whether we are on a *petanque* court or a soccer field, the *boule* or the soccer ball naturally exerts an attraction on us. We perceive it as an animated reality, a playing and even a challenging partner, which urges us to pick it up, bounce it, let it linger in our hands, and release it with a throw.[13] Holding the boule or the ball or any similar round, firm, and smooth object in our hands evokes in us, in the words of Buytendijk, a "feeling of cohesion (*Geschlossenheit*) without any resistance."[14] When taking a ball into our hands, we do more than sense its qualities; we also become aware of our own way of feeling ourselves. We feel an inner peace and calm while gently caressing its surface and taking pleasure in its stability and consistency. Once we release it, the ball seems to exploit its own resources and its full possibilities to move as if it wanted both to follow the imparted directive and to assert its own independence by disregarding, or at least modifying, the expected direction and position. If this unpredictability were missing in the moving ball, we would never spend so much time playing with it; nor would we likely ever go to watch players who excel in ball-handling.

Beyond their technical mastery, participants in ball games are repeatedly surprised by the movement of a ball when it deviates from what they have planned and expected. Beginners and expert players know that an unusually spectacular throw or kick, resulting in flawless execution, requires more than the technical and tactical skills acquired over a long period of training. It is an unpredictable achievement that eludes reflexive control and careful calculation. Surprising winning points are often scored when players, with an attitude of unconcerned surrender, allow their bodily impulses and powers to organize the movements and take care of the ball's release. Conversely, unexpected failures also happen when the legs or hands – or even the ball itself – trump the conscious control of movements. It is just such surprising moments, scoring or failing to score a goal, that make a game an enjoyable and even memorable experience for spectators and players alike.

Certain animals perceive the possibilities contained in a ball just as well as we do. Merely confronted by a flat piece of paper on the floor in front of it, a cat will not move. But once the paper is transformed into a ball, the feline, seeing the form's motor possibilities, immediately starts to play with it. In its new form, the paper "comes alive" and, as an image, suggests the possibility of tossing it around and running after it. As Hans-Georg Gadamer accurately observed: "The cat at play chooses the ball of wool because it responds to play, and ball games will be with us forever because the ball is freely mobile in every direction, appearing to do surprising things of its own accord."[15]

Beyond our playful interaction with an animated reality, a pathic encounter exposes us to something that unexpectedly occurs, something that we did not foresee and that we welcome with emotions ranging from joy or sorrow: an unfortunate turn of events, a happy coincidence, a chance happening, a missed encounter. Those taking part in sports competitions or live musical performances or journeying through a far-flung land inevitably enter situations or undertake activities that remain open-ended and trigger surprising plot twists. Various public spectacles and contests (the Tour de France, for instance) consist of a search for the smooth realization of a planned continuity in the face of a threat of disequilibrium, disorganization, and even chaos. Yet one of their appeals consists precisely in what we find in great novels: the pathic tension and astonishment maintained by the momentous surprises that, one after another, suddenly belie all tentative expectations.

Buytendijk speaks of the "pathic existence" (*pathische Existenz*) originating in a child's innocent and inspired play.[16] Its initial manifestation is an attachment to animated realities, a sympathetic and imaginative communication with the language of forms. The child takes two pieces of wood glued together and plays with them *as if* they were an airplane. Adopting the attitude of a pilot while flying on a toy airplane presupposes a dual, ambiguous relation to things: an objective relation to the pieces of wood seen as material and practical realities, and an emotional bond to extended forms as they display their manifold possibilities and appealing animated traits.[17]

Let us consider an everyday and early expression of the pathic existence in relation to animated forms. In his essay entitled "Child's Play," Robert Louis Stevenson recalls some of the cherished memories of his childhood. When he and other "right-minded children" were called to together for their meals, they felt that they must "find some imaginative sanction" to "colour," to "render entertaining," and to "enliven" the process of eating and drinking. His cousin poured sugar on the porridge and saw in this phenomenon a country buried under snow; he, in turn, poured milk on his food and viewed it as an island under the menace of gradual inundation.[18] The food, "seasoned with dreams," received a new significance and the process of eating became an unfolding imaginary life-story. Beyond the pleasure felt in presence of such a "phenomenal transubstantiation," the children discovered the referential quality of the objects. Not only did they turn to their otherwise unsavoury food with "furious interest" and succeed in creating a relation of affective intimacy with it, but they also realized that sugar and porridge, porridge and milk, in their animated forms – snow, island, sea – were, one might say, in a relation of kinship with each other. The pathic attitude perceives forms as animated realities and recognizes the same natural and magnetic attraction between them as exists between the dancer and the music, the player and the ball.

An emotional relation to animated realities presupposes a sensitive body that grasps the expressive and dynamic structure of things and their alluring relation to each other, and accomplishes an imaginative motor response in accordance with "elaborate stories of enchantment." In this respect, Hubertus Tellenbach has rightly emphasized the central role that the "pathic body," endowed with a "pathic sensibility," plays in human life.[19] Children react to early impressions through their "pathic body" and, at later stages of their lives, develop corresponding emotional reactions and dispositions toward pleasant or painful experiences. These experiences and the suitable pathic responses become "decisive criteria" for the course and distinctive characteristics of each person's life history. They remain inscribed on the living body, which, in the words of Gabriel Marcel, is a "temporal form."[20] The sensitivity of the body, formed over time through manifold experiences, gives significance to all sorts of realities, recognizes situations that are relevant, and creates a relation of dynamic reciprocity between significance and situation. Following the reflections of Tellenbach, we can assert that the playful view of life, developed in our childhood, defines to some extent the ways we relate to everyday realities in our adulthood – to our work, family, health issues, leisure activities, and love relations.

In the story related by Stevenson and his cousin, repeated tactile contacts between the spoon and the food create both a relation of intimacy and an enchanting merriment at table. A meal that is not touched, smelled, tasted, chewed, and swallowed is just as meaningless as an unread novel or an unperformed symphony. The pathic transformation of the significance of food is enacted mainly by the sense of touch. Take, for instance, the child who puts his fingers on one of the cookies placed on the table and emphatically cries out: "It's mine, I have already touched it." The indifferent thing becomes, in a magical fashion, an exclusive and cherished possession. In a child's life, the contrast between familiar and foreign, private and public, living and dead, animated and inanimate, direct and evasive, present and absent realities is established by the sense of touch. Before such a distinction is made, the familiar objects around them exhibit their expressive and trusted presence and solicit the approaching movement of the hand. While being touched and played with, these objects speak to the child and elicit loving and caring forms of behaviour. A doll above all, and also a pebble, a shell, a leaf, or feather, conveys to his or her hands the significance of a living and responsive reality. Independently of their material appearance, these things reveal to the child, especially when they are touched, their lovable, alluring, enthralling, and even vulnerable aspects.[21]

As adults, we adopt the same pathic attitude when we gently handle a valued book, a treasured tool, or an old car, and express our emotional attachment to these objects through the movement of our hand. Beyond the fondness we feel for such objects, we also value the pathic experience itself, the hand's gentle and playful embrace of the object. Giving up a favourite musical instrument, a piano for example, implies the loss of tactile contact with a familiar object. It was perhaps this same feeling of loss that led the writer Charles Lamb to confess the following after his retirement: "My old desk; the peg where I hung my hat, were appropriated to another. I knew it must be, but I could not take it kindly."[22]

In the absence of this kind of intimacy, people seek and relish tactile contact with other objects; they feel the need to hold a coffee cup, a cell phone, a pencil, a notebook, a set of keys; they fiddle with their tie or scarf, or repeatedly arrange their hair or gently caress their shaved chin or their beard. They seem to be searching for a momentary or lasting contact with something that fills the emptiness of their hands and provides an occasion to adopt, often unknowingly, an attitude of play. Those who attempt to quit smoking see themselves deprived of the exciting and nervous play of their fingers with a pleasurable object.

A similar play of the hands appears in gambling. In one of his widely read short stories, Stefan Zweig describes how the playing hands express the addicted gamblers' whole personality and obsession.[23] The story suggests that addiction to roulette in a casino can be illustrated in part by a gambler's dependence on the extraordinary vitality of the hands. Gamblers learn to exert strict control over their facial expressions; they "wear a cold mask of impassivity." And because they concentrate their attention on keeping every movement of their face in check, they forget, as they wait for the fall of the ball, how the spontaneous and individual movements of their hands or the way they hold and place the chips "shamelessly reveal their innermost secrets." The story brings into focus not merely the "impassioned expressiveness" of the great variety of hands, but also, and perhaps chiefly, the pathic lure created by the act of gambling itself. As an observer, a middle-aged woman becomes absorbed in the spectacle of heightened tensions, surprises, reliefs, and reversals; she is taken by the atmosphere of excitement generated by the alternation of loss and gain, the ebb and flow of passions. With an unconcerned and self-forgetting attitude, she immerses herself in the game; the sounds, movements, and gestures that contrast with the dispassionate glances, and thereby faithfully reflect the players' feelings, hold her spellbound. With curiosity she watches the exalted life, the "expressive eloquence" of a unique pair of "speaking hands." Each of them induces a spontaneous valuation, because each of them expresses distinct habits, passions, and affective reactions, moving from illusion to disillusion or to satisfaction according to the whim of the roulette wheel. And finally, she feels strangely drawn not only to a pair of magical hands and an intense and fascinating face, but to a human being in his totality and to all the risks that such an unforeseen encounter with a mysterious "young man of perhaps twenty-four" inevitably entails.

Pathic responsiveness to an animated reality, to a surprise, to a chance encounter, to what unexpectedly happens to someone, is the central element of a widely shared experience – the unfolding of a love-relationship.[24] Such singular moments often happen early in life, around the age of puberty. Perhaps it is the change in the inflection of the voice, a slight stress in the word of greeting, a furtive smile, an enquiring gaze, or a half-finished sentence that creates the impression of "love at first sight."[25] In the first stages of falling in love, one is inclined to adopt a playful attitude, though less consciously because of the novelty of the experience and perhaps for no other reason than to mitigate the force of the emotions. According to C.S. Lewis, in his illuminating and enlivening book on love, Venus demands from sensitive lovers total and immediate surrender, and this "is the very reason for preserving always a hint of playfulness in our attitude to her."[26] The pathic attitude of play, responding more carefully to a charming gaze or a mellifluous voice, produces a dual result: it pulls someone toward another person and, at the same time, presents ways of resisting love's intoxicating power. By conversing with someone playfully, making humorous remarks, asking confusing questions, not letting the other finish a sentence, a person lets the other obliquely know that he or she refuses to succumb to the loss of self-control portended by the surging feelings. The exchange of first glances, of smiles, of initial whispers, and later the touching of hands, are all marked by the fluctuation of feelings: doubt, reticence, hesitation, excitement, interest succeed each other.

It is the mutual hesitation and feeling of uncertainty that makes falling in love different from flirtation. Two persons flirting with one another choose to take on a playful attitude – and I shall return to this later – and, at a same time, hold on to the inner resolution not to fall in love, to stop short of committing themselves to an earnest and intimate relation. The amorous person lacks this kind of determination to lead another person on and communicate misleading promises. Conversation is occasionally transformed into rambling and meandering exchanges and may seem to show no progress at all; yet the partners implicated resonate even to tedious platitudes and respond to all dull or exciting communicative elements by guessing whether a further advance or a momentary retreat is the more judicious step to take. Just as in a play situation, they live with the need to make timely choices and the obligation of facing uncertainty; they are moved by words, intonations, and gestures and called to react to every verbal or nonverbal clue accordingly. They are like a seismograph – acutely sensitive and responsive to the slightest tremors.

Beyond initial surprise and the ensuing uncertainty, ambiguity is another characteristic aspect of an encounter prompted by emerging desires. This is eminently present in the feelings of the partners involved in an encounter; they are as charmed as troubled by the unexpected exchange with a new person in their lives. The ambiguity reveals itself first in the glance, which communicates both openness and concealment, as well as sympathy and reserve. One of the possible responses to a desiring glance is the mutual blush, which expresses neither consent nor rejection, but more the surprise of being happily affected by the presence of the other and the corollary wish to hold the surging feeling in check.

Words uttered in a tone of warm playfulness elicit spontaneous smiles that reassert the will to both create closeness and keep one's distance, which in turn intensifies uncertainty and ambiguity. Thanks to the remarkable malleability, mobility, and individuality of the face, a smile is capable of conveying a great number of nuances. Since each part of the face affects the whole, all these nuances come across vividly. A slight movement of the mouth blends into the rest of the face. Scintillating eyes give the impression of a radiant look; a sombre gaze creates a gloomy mien. As Helmuth Plessner pointed out, a smile implies a relaxation of the face and "in relaxing, the face offers itself as a field of play."[27] When roaring with laughter, a person is carried away by his or her overpowering emotion. "In smiling, on the other hand, there is a poised relationship to oneself and the world; the smile permits the face *playfully* to exhibit something."[28] A smile can also assume the function of a mask. And behind that mask there can be restraint, daring, calm tenderness, confident insistence, vacillation or decisiveness; the partners play with the protective distance created by a smile: they take a step forward, yet they remain elusive. Whatever remains hidden behind the mask, a smile still tells something, prompts questions about its meaning, offers a field for playful guessing, and keeps alive the pathic bond to the leisurely evolving love affair. Beyond all its possible shades and interpretations, a smile may also be animated, without any reserve, by the feeling of genuine gentleness. In such instances, it illuminates the whole being of the person, and the perception of this singular expression warms the heart, then fills one with relaxed confidence and exuberance.

The slight touch of the hands, the caress of other parts of the body, and kissing are all expressive acts that bring to the fore the pathic aspect of an encounter and call upon a play attitude. Under the impulse of sincere desire, lovers' hands initiate their own playful conversation, during which they are both moving and being moved, expressing the presence of the whole person and the love felt by one for another. Equally, the delicate caress of the hands, arms, shoulders is not merely a search for pleasurable contact with the body as flesh but the expression of the desire to reach for the animated presence of the person through his or her body. Playful hand movements stress the spiritual, the elevating aspects of love while at the same time responding to the pathic appeal created by the partner's body.

Lovers admit, though, that in the initial stage of their amatory encounter, they do not really know what to say or what to do. As in other situations that require confidence and ease for taking the first steps, the arrival of a playful attitude can in no small measure dispel tension by introducing humour and laughter, and – along with the language of the hands – temporarily deflect attention from the full expression of their physical desire for intimacy. Lovers should yield to Lewis's advice: "We must not attempt to find an absolute in the flesh. Banish play and laughter from the bed of love and you may let in a false goddess."[29] The false goddess may appear in the form of rigid and selfish behaviour that tends to degrade an intimate encounter to the level of a lust-fuelled biological event and fails to refer to any deeper feeling or value, missing altogether the central element of genuine bodily love: spiritual affinity with the whole person. In so doing, the partners view the body in its pure material reality, as a sort of tool, rather than as a symbol through which the persons, in their uniqueness, become present in the act of giving themselves to each other. The false goddess forbids jokes and laughter, especially in those initial moments when lovers are surprised by their nervousness, clumsiness, and, sometimes, indisposition to love. The contradiction between the remarkable aptness and astonishing awkwardness of the bodies, their graceful yet gawky form and movement, caused Lewis to compare lovemaking to buffoonery: "Lovers, unless their love is very short-lived, again and again feel an element not only of comedy, not only of play, but even of buffoonery, in the body's expression of Eros."[30]

Lewis also refers to a less frequent aspect of the intimate encounter: experiencing desire and, for the time being, receiving no satisfaction and feeling like a fool. "She (Venus) is a mocking, mischievous spirit, far more elf than deity, and makes games of us. When all external circumstances are fittest for her service she will leave one or both the lovers totally indisposed for it."[31] Lovers who admit that Venus is not subject to control and take her capricious withdrawal lightly will make jokes about it and even burst out in laughter. Because, as Lewis so wisely put it: "It is all part of the game; a game of catch-as-catch-can, and the escapes and tumbles and head-on collisions are to be treated as a romp."[32] Tomfoolery and laughter are, then, salutary responses to a situation in which the anticipation of delight meets no realization.

The other aspect of lovers' intimacy – doubtless much more frequently encountered – is the relaxed and pleasurable responsiveness of the partners in lovemaking. Here desire meets its full realization, including the play of love (what Jan Linschoten calls the "song of desire"), and, while scaling the heights of pleasure, the lovers meet each other as persons. Without much thinking, they know that love without play is something sombre and sad.[33]

There seems to be no consensus about the value of this obvious aspect of a fulfilling encounter between two lovers, experienced by countless persons of all ages. Some serious-minded yet not necessarily gloomy philosophers tend to address the phenomenon of sexual love by ignoring or neglecting the participants' play attitude. In Roger Scruton's detailed investigation of sexual desire, for instance, the reader finds no comment or discussion about saying silly things, tickling, or giggling in bed. In her review of the book, Martha Nussbaum justly reproaches Scruton for never saying that sexual desires and encounters can be fun. Yet lovers find delight in teasing each other in bed, in laughing wholeheartedly, and in relying merrily, in a state of utter absence of constraint, on the "improvisatory freedom" of their bodies.[34] Over hundreds of pages, the philosopher Scruton has tried to transpose into a rational sphere a human experience that is much larger than this sphere. Its motives and concrete expressions cannot be grasped by rational thinking alone. The vantage point of a loving person is not the same as the viewpoint of a rational thinker. The latter submits the subject matter to impersonal and reasoned judgments, whereas the former is involved in an intimate, personal experience in which affective, sensual, and imaginative communication plays a central role. Remy Kwant put the matter very well when he said: "the attitude which a person assumes when he considers this topic rationally is very different from the attitude of a married couple in their sexual togetherness."[35]

In this context, "improvisatory freedom" consists of moving without conscious control, letting the body propose the suitable approach or response, not following any previously elaborated representation. It calls for an unconcerned and relaxed surrender to the body's singular potential for invention, variation, and adventure. Just as in dancing, the partners abandon themselves to the natural spontaneity of their bodies. Without purposeful pre-assessment or planning, they delicately modify their gestures and invent surprising and unusual movements. In this, they are pathically guided by their own feelings, their own movements, and, above all, by the amorous responses of their partner. Their improvisatory spontaneity then allows them to achieve what usually eludes them in their daily lives; namely, the experience of alert relaxation of, and pleasurable unity with, their bodies. Pathic encounters between two playful partners may be regarded as a premonition of the possibility of achieving synchrony, with or without utilitarian considerations, on other levels of human existence. The resulting sense of agreement felt with one's own body is also amenable to the achievement of a similar spontaneous and attentive surrender to the demands and calls of a wider reality: a home, a neighbourhood, a city, or a natural environment.

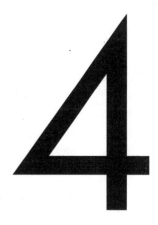

Ease

et us go to a public park on a luminous Sunday afternoon and watch children gambolling, throwing balls to each other, sitting on see-saws pushing up with their legs, or building a bridge in a sandbox over a long ditch filled with water. Their movements may be slightly awkward; they happen to drop the ball or miss their target; they see their construction collapsing and undertake urgent repairs before bringing another pail of water. But all these actions are carried out with astonishing ease and without apparent physical effort. Children seem to invent words and gestures, and imitate all the tasks and actions of any given profession faithfully, seriously, and without any constraint. And in play in which they occasionally have to remain immobile and wait for their turn to act, they may achieve quietness and self-awareness. One thinks of the game of staring into each other's eyes without blinking or laughing, or the graveyard game requiring participants to lie immobile on the ground as if they were lifeless. The obligation to *not* act – not move, not laugh, not speak, not make any noise – may be seen as a positive act: it is the task that players have to perform. The recent Mindball Game, in which the aim is to move a ball with one's brainwaves, reveals that the winner is the one who is more focused and relaxed. What is it that gives children the immediate sense of ease and stillness to be able to transform their world according to their desires and ideas, at the same time as facilitating their mutual interaction with each other?

We have seen earlier that in play we establish a changed set of relations to the objects of our everyday world. By a sort of magic, objects become animated things, communicating a distinct language and appearing with transformed qualities; everyday usages, customs, conventions, and behaviour no longer – or only partially – apply. The players become "magicians" who free objects from their habitual significance and their usual role in our familiar world. They move into another world where life acquires a new and distinctive mode of being. The usual tensions and obligations that arise from our habitual social interactions in private and public worlds cease to exert their influence. In speaking of this "suspension of the ordinary," Kenneth L. Schmitz observed: "The world of play with its own non-natural objectives and formalities may be said to transcend the natural world and the world of everyday concern."[1] Players assume a new sense of self when they become immersed in the to-and-fro experience that, as in all play, is tied to no decisive goal whose achievement would bring the experience to an end. Hence, clearly, the ease with which the players hold to the demands of play and keep alive their play-spirit.

We recall that play is characterized by a relation of reciprocity with something that, because of its mobility and expressive quality, sends an "appeal" to play and then plays with whoever receives the invitation. Because players are *drawn into* play, they are relieved from the task of taking the initiative; they enter play and pursue their activities as participants. We know from experience that, in accomplishing a goal-oriented obligation in a work setting, the distance we walk requires more exertion than the same distance would require if we were walking with no purpose, seeking only the pleasure of absorbing the manifold impressions around us in an unconcerned state of mind. In leisurely situations we are pulled by our captivating surroundings as if connected by an invisible cord. Erwin Straus's conclusions on the difference between purposive movement and dance movement, and between energy expenditures in goal-oriented, directional spaces and in non-directed, acoustically rich spaces apply also to the experience of playful activities.[2] In many forms of play, just as in dance, our movements respond either to the structure of the space we are in, without any direction, or to an object free of goal-oriented intention. A sense of freedom and of being connected with one's surroundings, as well as our full absorption in the pleasurable activity, induces and prolongs the experience of playful ease.

We also observe, however, that in some forms of play, the kind of pleasurable pathic participation in activity that results in the dissolution of subject-object tension is not fully achieved. When players seek to maintain a distance in respect to the object and partner of play, they don't let the activity carry them away fully. There are forms of play that call for clear thinking and detached imagining about making and changing rules, the relation between means and end, the modification of ends with respect to means, and, conversely, the modification of means with respect to new ends. Such activities give players the possibility of exploring new ways of playing and of inventing entirely new forms of play. They also provide occasions to relate to play in a flexible manner, to take pleasure in an experience of relative freedom in thinking and imagining that can lead to a sense of lightness and openness.

A distinction among diverse forms of play caught the attention of Eugen Fink. He correctly observed that in role-playing games, individuals can identify themselves with their characters to such an extent that they lose their own distinctive personality. They forget themselves and, as it were, "sink into a role." A self-forgetful and dream-like state such as this helps a player move and speak with minimum constraint. In role-playing, the adoption of a genuine play attitude endows one's movements with the appearance of natural grace. "The play can imply a more profound, almost unconscious performance; it can also be approached with a lighter hand and a gracefully floating elegance."[3] There are, on the other hand, plays of pretending in which the participants deal with their character with stiffness, a sense of control; they are careful to uphold a reflexive distance towards their actions.

Doing something with ease and dexterity is often the result of an expertise gained after a long period of strenuous practice. Musicians, dancers, or athletes have developed both habit and skill. Habit grants them facility, skill proficiency. For them playfulness consists in their ability to disguise the long period of repetitive learning behind the appearance of effortlessness. They bring together both unflinching will and graceful ease.

Genuine experts do not always seek to surpass themselves when they excel in their art. Time and again they propose a work of a lesser magnitude than their creative faculties would allow them to achieve. Many conceive and create something by intentionally not exploiting their admirable aptitudes to the hilt, by not using all the resources of their spiritual and bodily abilities. In such cases, the transcendence of which Schmitz speaks takes an altered form in the creative act. Some artists, for instance, are able to take a critical distance from their own talent, as well as from their hard-won knowledge and expertise, and make decisions with regard to the degree to which they apply their skills and ideas. The restraint they impose on themselves when they speak, write, act onstage, or carve a wooden figure, for instance, gives them both freedom and a sense of leisure. They relate to their text or other type of artistic material with playful ease, never with strenuous effort.

Holding back something within, such artists exhibit to a remarkable degree the virtues of reserve, modesty, and discretion that are captured by the French term *litote*. *Litote*, the ability to hold a creative power in check and exercise restraint, is the guarantor of lightness, immediacy, refinement, and liveliness in whatever one decides to create. It even promises something more. Michel Serres goes as far as to state: "Possessing a power and not using it, this is the beginning of wisdom. And of civilization."[4] In relation to children's games, Serres observed that *litote* consists of reducing with facility everything large to a small scale. G.K. Chesterton proposes a similar ethical and aesthetic principle in his "philosophy of toy theatre": "Art does not consist of expanding things. Art consists of cutting things down, as I cut down with scissors my very ugly figures of St. George and the Dragon."[5]

One thinks also of the experience of the lightness and ease of amateur musicians, who are free from the imperative to faultlessly execute a musical work; they play their chosen pieces for the pleasure of playing. They seem to appreciate the possibility of playfully setting aside the conventions and obligations of professional standards and, confidently relying on the availability and spontaneity of their bodies, bringing subtle ornamentations and slight deviations into their playing. In trusting the capabilities of their own bodies and adopt a play attitude, they perceive their task, instruments, and surroundings less as things to be confronted and mastered than as a support and a wellspring of pleasure in playing. By actively taking on an attitude of play and maintaining it, amateurs can create or strengthen an emotional relationship with their milieus and to some extent shape and transform these milieus.

A change in our customary way of experiencing our body in its environment can intensify the sensation of ease. Let us consider for a moment our experience of swimming for pleasure, without any need to achieve technical perfection or reach a goal. The change becomes apparent when we abandon our vertical posture, which, although natural, requires constant effort, and relax into a horizontal position, as happens when we swim unhurriedly in a lake or a pool. As we enter the water, we enjoy a new kind of relationship with the world through the repetition of our spontaneous and easy-flowing motions. Just as lying in bed induces the feeling that we are not facing an objective world and are, as it were, reconciled with a warm and comfortable environment, swimming brings about a similar feeling: the tension between the self and the objective world melts away in the experience of floating. We become one with the play of waves. In water, we enjoy the sense of being carried, a kind of buoyancy, as we seemingly defy the laws of gravity. We welcome a freedom unknown to our everyday existence, as our arms and legs move without restraint. We give ourselves to the delightful feeling of weightlessness and become keenly aware of a sense of ease and relief from obligations and concerns. Hannah Arendt, relating her experience of free movement in the Aegean Sea in a letter to her mentor and lifelong friend Karl Jaspers, rejoices in this sense of ease: "Whenever I can, I go swimming. Swimming always gives me a feeling of being at home."[6]

What makes Arendt feel so much at home in the sea? I have already mentioned that one's attitude determines the experienced qualities of one's immediate surroundings. The wish to perform an action playfully springs from the desire to be keenly aware of our own being and, at the same time, the wish to establish a new relationship with the surrounding world. Through the lived movements and the pathic attraction of a milieu, we have the potential to transform a quantitative, abstract, natural, and prosaic surrounding into a qualitative, concrete, human, and poetic medium.[7] One possible result of a play attitude is to transform matter and its meaning through a creative act. When we swim, we inhabit our lived space in water, the meaning of which is defined by the pleasurable movement we enjoy in it. Swimming, therefore, may be seen as an act of connection and organization whereby water adapts itself to our movements, creating a synthesis between our body and the world.

When we walk, paddle, or ski playfully, we may share Arendt's contentment and say to ourselves, "I am now in my element." We celebrate a feeling of intimate unity with our milieu, which presents itself with qualities of warmth, friendliness, and availability, and with the aesthetic values that we cherish. To feel "at home" somewhere, in a public library or in a forest meadow, is to feel no tension between ourselves and our surroundings.

While interacting with trees and flowers as we see, smell, or touch them, we establish these sensory relations calmly, unhurriedly, without constraint, and find sources of harmony and rest in these newly animated realities. The restful relation we create is reminiscent of the effects of such acts as contemplating an alpine meadow or listening to a Mozart *Andante*, which offer us the possibility of being peacefully absorbed in what we perceive and finding tranquillity and inspiration.[8]

I have mentioned the primary conditions for bringing an attitude of playful ease into our lives. This ease manifests differently in the activities that we accomplish, according to our level of proficiency. Entering a communal dance calls for a different degree of ease than is helpful for conducting a difficult negotiation. There is, of course, a huge difference between the facility with which a child's hands randomly hit piano keys and the ease and articulation with which an accomplished performer's fingers perform a musical composition – even though both may enjoy an intimacy with the instrument and both adopt a pathic attitude to the sounds. For the skilled musician, ease comes after a long period of study and practice, thanks to the adoption of a self-forgetting and relaxed attitude toward his or her performance; for the child, facility is the gift of his or her natural, unaffected, uninhibited way of acting and being.

There is a German term for the attitude of ease that musicians, dancers, and athletes, as well as children may experience; it is not much used today in everyday conversation and is rather difficult to translate: *Unbefangenheit*.[9] It connotes an inner freedom, the freedom of not being inhibited or constrained by thought, a feeling of not being held back by doubts, hesitations, or distrust – of not being confined by a bodily limitation. Fearing danger – being intimidated by the magnitude of a perceived risk – is among the concerns that can weigh heavily on a person and create an unwelcome constraint. The words and actions of an unconstrained person are direct, carefree, and spontaneous. We can observe the fully engaged attitude of children when they handle their toys and dedicate themselves to their activities with no concern for the opinions of onlookers. The environment they are surrounded by is responsive, full of animation. In this space, they are invited to become what they are playing: to sing as an instrument would sing, to fly as a toy airplane would fly.

A similar mimetic attitude is characteristic of those who engage in the banter of a pub or market place. They show no concern at all for the life buzzing around them or for the trajectory of time in its irrevocable forward movement. They turn to their fellow human beings in a state of complete self-forgetfulness and with a willingness to create a common understanding through the mirroring of each other's words and gestures. The imitative repetition of greetings, banalities, congratulations, interjections, exhortations, exchanges of news, pieces of advice, complaints, or qualms over doubtful statements follow each other with vivacity and genuine naturalness.

Lively chatter is spontaneous – neither calculated and artificial nor strained and mannered. It takes place without cautious reflection or elaborate reasoning. Its words and gestures have no functional or utilitarian value. The interlocutors relate to each other with trust and without any "hidden agenda." Sudden and even impulsive comments, exclamations, objections, and agreements emerge with direct, dynamic, and prompt expression. Questions and answers, following each other closely and with unconstrained ease and no deliberate preparation, seem to arise from fertile and unknown layers of the body.

In referring to these deep bodily resources, which, of course, shape more than our enjoyable and leisurely conversations, the French philosopher René Le Senne spoke of a "superabundance of energy" intermingling with our will, and of a "generous exuberance, giving without reckoning the cost and never economizing."[10] Le Senne called this spontaneity naïve, "because it comes to us as a gratuitous gift which we have only to accept with ingenuousness."[11] Our surrender to the wealth of "inner powers," which carry us along and out of which movements, words, and ideas effortlessly burst forth, is a common characteristic of many activities.[12] In this respect, a child's running and jumping is as spontaneous as the movements of a dancer who proposes an unusual combination of gestures or of an artist who, dexterously and without any planning, allows a hand to propose a surprising modification of a painted or sculpted form. Notwithstanding the different degrees of preparation and skill that each of these activities requires, the child, the dancer, and the artist are united in their shared experience of delight and ease. According to Le Senne, the same "ingenuous intoxication" can be found in all such manifestations of joy in life, creativity, and artistic innovation.[13]

Unconstrained human interactions of this sort bring forth a relation of reciprocity characteristic of trustful and disinterested collaboration and unperturbed exchanges of ideas. The trust granted to a child or a colleague generates an atmosphere of free interaction and, correspondingly, an ambience in which everyone can speak and move with ease. This atmosphere quickens a culture of open collaboration and mutual aid. We remember fondly those of our teachers who began their classes with a few humorous remarks and playful riddles and succeeded in putting dazzling smiles on their students' faces. The relaxed atmosphere, created in all sincerity by the teacher, fosters a relation of confidence and esteem, and spawns heightened curiosity and whetted interest in the subject.

I suspect that Lewis Thomas had this approach to education in mind when he recommended a departure from the habitual way of teaching scientific subjects. He suggested that teachers begin by focusing on what is not yet known, what is left to be discovered and explored, and, by calling students' attention to the mysteries and paradoxes of life on our planet, awakening in them a sense of puzzlement, curiosity, and fun. This encouragement to see science as a "high adventure" invites students to dispel the anxiety and tension that they would inevitably feel as the result of spending many a dreary hour in the library memorizing dry theories and lifeless facts – the so-called basics. By making the research endeavour appealing, guided by the admission of one's ignorance and the need for persistent questioning, Lewis succeeded in appropriately comparing the transformation of answers into questions to a "game" and saw in this game the condition of important scientific advances.[14] The extent to which students make this reverse mode of learning and doing research their own and keep tackling problems with a sense of curiosity and ease, substantiates Rudolf Arnheim's assertion: "I have come to believe that what students learn from their teachers is mainly the attitude behind teaching."[15]

Whether we seek to address new scientific problems in theory or to bring our expertise to the realization of a project in a concrete setting, we find ourselves energized by the prospect of collaboration in the absence of suspicion, envy, or any other sort of negative feeling. We realize that we are able, for a certain time at least, to express ourselves freely and respond to expectations without concern. We also notice that others relate to us with a similarly liberated mindset and gladly take part in conversations about science, urban design, or any other interest. Work shared with peers combines gentle teasing and humour with creative improvisations. If we stop and reflect on the reasons for experiencing such a pleasant and stimulating atmosphere, we might become aware that the people around us are inquisitive and enthusiastic as well as open and authentic; that they speak and act without any carefully crafted self-representation. Their words and deeds express directly what they think, want, and feel, without simulation or pretense.

"Conversation is only possible when men's minds are free from pressing anxieties,"[16] asserted Somerset Maugham when writing on the conditions suitable for writing good prose. It should, he said, resemble the conversation of persons enjoying free and leisurely interaction. William James shared this view, declaring that a conversation gives enjoyment when "people forget their scruples and take the brakes off their hearts."[17] We could apply these observations to other human endeavours in which overworry about the quality and consequences of actions or words makes people question themselves. The favourable outcome of an artistic undertaking, a scientific project, or a political negotiation depends largely on the participants' ability to banish doubts, hesitations, and anxieties about the future and to act in the present with confidence in the felicitous turn of events beyond their influence. Abandoning their concerns about the consequences of their decisions, they may succeed in creating a "sympathetic contact" with their current situation and confidently entrust themselves to the future.[18]

Freedom from anxiety and the ability to relate to others with ease are characteristics of one kind of play attitude. As we shall see in the next chapter, however, an anxiety that arises from the awareness of future uncertainties may motivate a person to seek the risk of undertaking a hazardous activity and, paradoxically, to confront an approaching danger with a free and unbuttoned attitude.

How do we imagine our lived future? Counting on the consistency of our habits and the reliability of the institutions around us, we expect the periodic return of events and actions that we have already experienced. Admitting, however, that even our most assured predictions can be thwarted, we also generally allow for the arrival of surprising events and unexpected changes. For some people, however, it is almost unbearable to face an unpredictable future with the possibility of unforeseen changes. Such people develop a defensive behaviour consisting of anticipating concrete adversities and cancelling out the possibilities of real fulfilling experiences. For them it is easier to deal with the realization of well-defined negative possibilities than with overpowering and at the same time elusive uncertainties. There are still others who close themselves against the future by refusing to consider even the slightest deviation from their well-established routines and well-trodden paths, and thus turn away from all the new possibilities arising in the present. As the past is extended, the present is narrowed, and the future approaches without any novelty or diversity. As a result, lived time loses its historical continuity.[19]

We adopt an altogether different prospective attitude when we let the future advance toward us with its wide-openness. We no longer count only on the foreseeable; we put aside the pursuit of certainties; we welcome surprising and unsuspected possibilities bestowed by the present; we take satisfaction in their realization even if they do not seem to open seamless and undisturbed paths. If we are willing to adapt our actions to current circumstances and not interfere with life's twists and turns, we will find ourselves able to undertake activities with lively grace, ease, and confidence. What is needed is the alacrity to look away from, and beyond, our cherished plans, to give up our deeply ingrained habits, and to remain receptive to new events and unforeseen encounters.

There is an element of playfulness in an attitude of non-attachment, in the readiness to change one's action and, to a certain extent, adjust a phase of one's life to the demands, suggestions, and invitations of circumstances as they arise. Of course, there is no question of playfulness in spontaneously helping a person in distress. But when we are not facing such a pressing call, we are able to act in numerous situations by following the clear intimations of the reality we encounter. One factor determining our inclination to accept what new situations suggest is our desire to heighten an expectative tension in ourselves, a feeling similar to what we experience while reading a detective story; our curiosity about the eventual outcome of our action is aroused. We have seen that playing consists of responding to the dynamic and sensory possibilities of an object. One can welcome and value this kind of momentary and spontaneous adaptation in artistic activities – theatre, painting, sculpture, dance, music – as well as in health care, education, politics, and even business and sport, when one becomes weary of the dictates of profitability and optimal performance. In all these domains, there is ample room for inventive improvisations consisting of the surprising introduction of more or less subtle deviations from a previously ensconced plan, script, strategy, or conception.

Unless severely constrained, we have the ability to accept the novelties that destiny holds in store for us and which make possible our positive response to those life-defining events that befall us unexpectedly and present us with unsettling uncertainties: a proposal to embrace an unsuspected professional career path, an invitation to move to an unknown city or country, or a call to depart from a habitual milieu and to join a community founded with a charitable purpose. Uncertainty about the prospects of our future existence can be welcomed with an attitude of play. We do not create the uncertainty, as we do in launching an adventurous business proposal; rather, the uncertainty comes to us and we encounter it in a state of composed curiosity.

Straus calls this attitude "serenity" – *Gelassenheit*.[20] He sees in the figure of Julius Caesar a model of the political leader who is able to entrust himself to the present moment and can surmount any difficulties encountered by undertaking "new and ingenious improvisations." Caesar conformed his actions to the circumstances that faced him and whatever knowledge was available in his present situation. His calm, serenity, and forbearance may have caused his downfall, says Straus, but these virtues also helped him attain greatness and celebrity. Caesar's serenity consisted in accepting his own limitations; while acting decisively and courageously, he allowed events to take their own due course; he lived by "letting things be."

Straus's reflections on the serene and poised attitude of Julius Caesar leads me to propose a few cursory remarks on what I hold as one of the main qualities of a leader. The idea of leadership, so attractive and yet so deleterious, has garnered ever-increasing attention in recent years. This trend has led to the publication of useful and stimulating works; but it has also advanced the false claim that everyone can be or should be an effective and successful leader, and that trumped-up and undisputed leaders gain a foothold only if they adopt a collegial attitude. Leaders who make daring decisions ultimately make them alone, even if they consult others first. Another completely fruitless idea holds that whoever proves to be an applauded champion in his or her field of expertise should be a leader. A leader is clearly someone who is able to survey a complex situation, analyze its chief elements, elaborate plans and strategies, make decisions, propose objectives and actions following a careful and rational assessment of a situation, create collaboration, set norms and values, evaluate the consequences of decisions, and react to emergencies with rapidity, timeliness, and decisiveness. In addition to possessing these qualities, leaders approach their activities, objectives, tasks, and duties with a consciously chosen attitude. There are leaders whose foremost aim is to serve themselves and promote their careers; and there are those who work relentlessly for just causes and the common good, and focus on bringing positive change into the lives of others. There are leaders who are overly active and are preoccupied with tangible results; others, although valuing efficiency and accomplishment, prefer to lead with an attitude of reposeful serenity. To my mind, the latter attitude consists not merely of conforming one's action to the suggestions or dictates of a situation but also of being able to delay an action or even not acting at all. A leader may prefer to not interfere – to postpone an action or let time take care of an issue by itself. This attitude of serenity in action means remaining in a state of expectation – taking a stance of not acting. Not acting can, in reality, be seen as an active and alert behaviour. The explicit obligation of not acting entails an implicit obligation to attentively wait until the moment is ripe for intervening.[21]

Tolstoy, in his novel *War and Peace*, saw General Mikhail Kutuzov's greatness in his simplicity and his ability to delay action: "Time and patience, these are my champions," the general reflected.[22] How should we understand the act of waiting? While waiting for a telephone call at home or for a medical examination in a health centre, we are ready to respond as soon as we hear the ring of the phone or the call of our name. We have to let some time pass in order to experience the expected and known event: the call. The passing of time is lived either in a state of acute tension or with calm resignation. Such waiting takes place in the present, which is marked by the expectation of a moment belonging to the immediate future. There is also another kind of waiting – a waiting that does not know what to expect from the future. We may see the future impetuously coming toward us and merely wait for this unknown future to become present and known. What does this unknown future hold for us? We may try to hold at bay an annihilating danger that fills us with anguish and exerts its inhibitive influence. Or we may think that something deeply satisfying will occur and we hasten its arrival through an effort of shrinking lived time with unceasing business. It is possible, however, to adopt another attitude toward the unknown future. We may turn to the future with easeful curiosity and inward tranquillity, with a playful state of mind. We allow the future to be "wide open," making no judgment about its fundamental fact and not forcing it to reveal what it will bring to the present. We let the future *play with us*, let it present its surprising proposal, question, or demand according to its pace and make us adapt to the rhythm and breadth of its disclosure with keenness and ease.

I believe that leaders of our time would benefit from a willingness to welcome the *play of the future*. They would achieve more if, occasionally, they were disposed to wait with relaxed serenity and repose, if they were ready to observe how future possibilities compete with each other until one of them reaches its realization. Then, while waiting in a state of comfortable serenity, they will be able to entrust themselves to the future and see that actions and interactions occur independently of their will and, in the fullness of time, will bring a happy resolution to present concerns. A serene attitude of this sort entails neither complete self-assurance nor relentless, hasty intervention in the affairs at hand. Serenity favours availability and adaptation, and withstands the pressure of an approaching future that seems to solicit action. It does not mean that leaders merely take their own time or refuse to commit themselves, and thus play for safety. "The serenity of a human being manifests itself in the style of welcoming things as they appear," wrote Bollnow, and this style affirms its superiority over harried activism.[23] Although serene leaders turn to the future with confidence and curiosity, the expectation of a particular outcome does not overshadow the present. Experience proves that, unless one encounters an emergency and is faced with the ineluctable obligation to act promptly, numerous contentious issues call for an attitude of non-activity untroubled by the passing of time, and an unworried attitude to the expected but still unknown outcome of a solution. In short, certain issues benefit from the practice of what Huxley called "the fine art of doing nothing."[24]

The mention of a "fine art" invites me to turn my attention to the quality of elegance. Elegance is a style that appears in unconstrained and graceful behaviour and finds its expression in a person's movement, speech, and conversation.[25] It comes into view when the participants of a game move with natural facility and shape their activity according to their individual capabilities and conceptions. Elegance is found in the acts of throwing a ball, dancing on ice, or climbing a mountain; the movements convey the impression of lightness and ease and, at the same time, they allow a glimpse of an implicit wealth of skills earned through strenuous practice. Elegant is the conductor whose direction indicates effortlessly, sparingly, yet with absolute precision, the desired tempo and the right shade of expression without excessively underscoring the depth of his comprehensive intimacy with the musical piece. Elegant is the teacher who brings to her students an erudition without affectation, who chooses the right tone, the most convenient words, and imparts the appropriate amount of knowledge. Elegance presupposes the ability to adopt, with keen sensitivity, the suitable response, the apt verbal style, the right approach to a problem.[26]

The art of choosing (*eligere*) is the starting point for the manifestation of elegance (*elegantia*). Elegant lecturers select the right amount of information to impart or things to describe, analyse, reflect upon, and question. The lectures of Aldous Huxley in *The Human Situation* serve as a good example. Huxley exhibits a wide range of penetrating insights and predictions – on such vital issues as the environment, violence, population growth, relation between private and public life, immediate and distant goods – reduced to their accessible essentials. If, as he put it, the function of literary persons is to build bridges between art and science, facts and values, abstractions and immediate experiences, elegant lecturers are builders of the bridge between the depth of assimilated knowledge and the restraint adopted while putting views across.[27]

"Elegance," asserted José Ortega y Gasset, "is marked by sobriety in plenitude. The capacity to obtain the maximum achievement with the minimum means."[28] In an elegant political speech, teaching style, wide-ranging conversation, or humorous story, we find a harmonious and delicate equilibrium between the force and exuberance appropriate to the expected effects and the suitability and subtlety of restraint in the means applied. The difficulty consists in knowing to what extent the reduction in the use of means yields the most favourable result, when the least brings forth the most, and when simplicity succeeds in conveying the highest values. One cannot apply a previously formulated rule to achieve the right span; the concrete circumstances dictate, in part at least, the appropriate realization of this paradoxical relation.

Calligraphy offers a particularly good illustration of the right balance sought and reached between exuberant inventiveness and disciplined mastery. Here, as Jean Lacoste has pointed out, the elegant movement of the calligraphic brush "succeeds in satisfying the contradictory requirements of construction and play."[29] Indeed, the exercise of calligraphy may be considered a form of play and the harmonious integration of purposive readability and aesthetic ornamentation is achieved thanks to the adoption of an attitude of play. A similar elegance is visible when an object – a door, a chair, or a weapon – conveys the fruitful reconciliation of the taste for ornament and the need for functional convenience. If we emphasize one at the expense of the other, the elegance is lost. In an elegant solution we detect a judiciously tempered force that "handles the difficulties with mastery and ease" and "ignores the resistance of an instrument and of a material."[30]

The elegance of the tennis player Roger Federer brings together the fluidity of his brilliant technique, the economy of his energy, and the simplicity of his gestures. I have just observed that choice presides over what a person manifests and says and what is held back and kept in reserve. How can someone make a choice with regard to a bodily initiative or a response in the heat of a moment? Hugo Rahner affirmed that the "shimmering elegance of some acquired skills" is attained only when "the gesture has been made obedient and pliable to the spirit."[31] But elegance is achieved also when the spirit has been made pliable to the gesture. The choice, then, has become fully integrated within the person and is therefore not consciously made before acting. There is simply no time for the survey of available options. A game of tennis becomes elegant, proficient, and seemingly effortless when the accomplished player comes to trust the indwelling intelligence of the body, and lets the hand swing, ignoring the dictates of the spirit. The virtuoso pianist's hands execute complex rhythmic figures with magisterial ease and introduce subtle expressive ornaments to each phrase with elegance when the urge to voluntary determination is resisted and yields to the natural spontaneity of the body and its already formed and learned skills. At the keyboard, such involuntary elegance obliterates difficulties and guarantees flawless execution. In its absence, the artist is prone to become stiff and make mistakes. Other sorts of gestures – especially those that spontaneously express benign impulses toward a fellow human being in a state of need – can also be elegant when they bypass the conscious will and rely only on the body's keen sense of rightness and proportion.

We find a happy marriage of playfulness and elegance when a task is approached in a relaxed way and does not require the use of all of our available powers. Elegant individuals undertake an activity with sensitivity, liveliness, naturalness, and ease and do not reveal all their inner resources and richness. Their achievements discreetly intimate the possession of an excess and undisclosed reservoir of creative energy. Thanks to the wealth of their inner worlds, they are poised to take up their task with both passionate engagement and light-hearted detachment. However significant and challenging a task may seem, such individuals approach it with sober elegance while maintaining a remarkable balance between adaptation and initiative, openness and restraint, passion and nonchalance. The mastery that they enjoy over their inner world and the conscious or unconscious choices they are able to make between what they express and what they conceal give a playful quality to their approach and make their execution appear effortless. They are able to adopt an attitude of play toward their own ideas and feelings as well as toward their activity in the moment.

Let us elucidate this relation to the self with a final illustration. An interview with significant personalities – authors, scholars, composers, actors – is elegant when the interviewed persons are able to choose spontaneously and with ease among the ideas and experiences they want to communicate, the details they want to delicately highlight, the questions they want cleverly to bypass or enthusiastically to address, the anecdotes they desire to tell. Successful interviews are enchanting, easy to follow, full of variety, and never stuffy or monotonous. Interviewed persons are skilled at revealing, without any affectation or false modesty, their unique and captivating personality and, at the same time, always telling less than they would be able to share. They possess an ability which, by definition, involves a perspective of distance toward the riches of their mind. This inner reflexivity gives them the freedom to choose among possible ways of communication and the playful facility with which to survey these possibilities and make use of one over another.

5

Risk

"The game of chance *(jeu de hasard)* is the soul of all games,"[1] wrote the French philosopher Alain, author of astute observations on play. Since ancient times, for children and adults alike, games of chance have been among the favourite types of play. They are played in a great variety of forms, according to a great variety of rules. Chief among them is the requirement to let luck and not conscious and deliberate choice or skill decide the outcome of the game. Luck is something that eludes foresight and control and determines an outcome favourable or unfavourable to the respective players. In all sorts of games, we are open to uncertain and uncontrollable happenings that bring us either a felicitous or an infelicitous result.

In the same way that we engage in games of chance without being able to influence the development and the results of our actions, so, in our everyday lives, we undertake activities whose outcomes are unpredictable and decided by "good" or "bad" luck. We encounter all kinds of people, from sympathetic colleagues and neighbours to friends and inspiring role models, to unpleasant and noisy travellers and harmful malefactors, by sheer luck. As we progress on the road of our becoming, we try to imagine and to predict the decisive moments of our life. Yet, notwithstanding careful planning, which surely brings stability into our daily existence and yields satisfactory experiences, we eventually come to realize that life-defining possibilities occur and meet us by happenstance, in states of uncertainty, and even force us to roll the dice of decision. In such situations, we preface our action by saying: "Let's see what happens if I undertake studies for an enthralling but poorly rewarded profession," or "What if I were to spend a year or two in a foreign place?" Or I might intentionally open myself to uncertainty: "If I decide to quit my unsatisfactory job, then numerous other alluring and unpleasant possibilities may open up for me," and then, perhaps, "If I select the possibility of creating a theatre company, I wonder what this daring venture will bring into my life."

Games of chance attract us because, in addition to the desire for material profit or the thrill of winning, we derive keen pleasure in surrendering to future uncertainties, correlating risks and counting on our good luck. "The attraction that the game exercises on the player lies in the risk," said Hans-Georg Gadamer.[2] We fancy playing with diverse possibilities and, once having freely committed to one possibility, we find ourselves anxiously or stolidly facing the alternatives: will we win or lose? Even when we participate in a simple playful activity such as building a sand castle, throwing a pair of dice, or placing a row of dominoes upright, we envisage intensely the possibilities of succeeding or of failing. The taste for living with risk, the desire to try our luck and allow good or bad fortune to come to us and put us to the test, finds its pleasurable expression in many elementary forms of play. The more a game requires the courage – or even the temerity – to take a risk, the greater the fascination it seems to exert on us.

I would define risk with regard to its effect on the temporal structure of our existence. When we take a risk, or when a risk falls upon us, we experience ourselves in relation to uncertainty and face the possibility of an undesirable experience. An awareness of risk implies that we survey our future possibilities in the act of estimating whether the eventual realization of one or several possibilities will bring us a favourable or an unfavourable outcome. Taking risks requires an attitude that involves foresight, speculation, and a partial or complete reliance on sheer chance. Even when an expected possible experience – the success or failure of a business venture in a foreign land, for instance – is still at a certain temporal distance from our present, the risk alters the way we live the present. When the awareness of risk enters the present, the seamless flow of segments of time from the "expected not yet" to the "realized now" is disturbed.

Let me try to convey this alteration of the present with an example. Suppose I were driving on a highway and sudden gust of freezing rain were to bring an unexpected risk to my otherwise monotonous travel – the risk of driving on a very slippery road and losing control over my car. If I assess the situation carefully and do not overly worry about the change in the road's condition and decide to continue my travel at a slower speed, my present is marked by the awareness of the possibilities of either continuing safely on the slippery road or being involved in an accident. I know quite well that I am not the only driver on this road and that another car, driven by a less careful individual, may hit my vehicle. I may keep on driving and respond to the peril I face with a certain apprehension or even with a feeling of excitement. I rely on my skill and my good luck in the presence of dangerous driving conditions. If, on the other hand, I decide to exit the highway and wait at the next stop-shop, I dispel from my lived present the possibility of experiencing a mishap. Concern about a disquieting possible future event no longer intrudes into my present; it is replaced by the less-troubling concern of arriving late at my destination. My way of turning to and evaluating future possibilities in the present leads me to take or to dodge the risk.

If I intentionally take the risk of continuing my travel on the slippery road, I become alert to the possible result of my decision. Since the outcome is obviously unknown, the risk entails either a heightened level of feeling or a state of complete indifference. I may undertake the risk like a gambler who, upon placing his chips on a colour and anticipating the outcome of the spin of the roulette wheel, experiences anxiety – and relishes it – for a short time. And this relished feeling is lived as a spur to action. The answer to his gamble comes quite quickly and, to recover the savoured emotional state, he has to repeat his bet. In many other risky undertakings – speculative activity on the stock exchange, for instance – the outcome becomes known only later, and the feeling of reward anxiety, whether dim or sharp, lasts longer.

As Heinz Heckhausen has shown in his study on play, even infants playing the game of covering their eyes with a blanket and experiencing the risk of bumping into an object and hurting themselves, are able to withstand – and even to seek – the tension of anxiety, if the temporal length of the experience does not exceed a certain limit.[3] Ernst Haigis, in his theory of play, sees the pleasure of experiencing "situations of vital endangerment" and the corresponding acceptance of startling risks as central motivating forces for undertaking playful activities. The agreeable sense of danger gives players a vivid awareness of their existence, the "blissful experience of 'I am.'"[4] And the overall experience of heightened self-awareness generates in the partici-pants a feeling of sympathy and a persistent attachment to the objects of play.

I may read in the newspaper about a volatile foreign currency, yet this distant prospect does not affect my life; I do not see this change in the value of a far-away currency as a risk for my own investments. On the other hand, the possibility of military confrontation between two heavily armed factions within my own city fills me with anxiety; I ask questions about the possible impact of the risk of war on my own life, my family, and my immediate sur-roundings. Any possible future experiences that concern us and play a role in our active lives are characterized by risk. The contingency planning that we do at home, at our workplace, or during travels reminds us that risks are at the heart of our existence. In fact, we live with uncertainty at every mo-ment of our existence; potential harms hover over us even if we do not think about them. We live with tacit risks insofar as our usual representation of the future is tied to the anticipation of both harmless and harmful possibilities. We live with the possibility of being hit on a road by a car or being deprived at home of vital resources for living such as electricity or water. Most of the time, we give so little weight to these kinds of risks that we come to ignore them or, if someone calls our attention to their presence, stoically put up with them. If, however, we attentively ponder what appear to us as more weighty risks (risks related to our health, for example), we attenuate their adverse or paralyzing effects by modifying our lifestyle or by adopting well-conceived countermeasures. Without being experts, we undertake a "risk analysis" of our living conditions, evaluate the eventual cost of mishaps or failings, and, if necessary, introduce new defensive measures according to possible future happenings. Nonetheless, eliminating the possibility of unwanted accidents from our lives is hardly conceivable, unless our becoming comes to a stand-still and the advance to the future is blocked by apathy, inactivity, or the inability to adequately adjust to changed circumstances.

Some people, assailed by the uncertainties of the future and unable to fore-see the consequences of their actions, are unwilling to take risks. One reason for their refusal is a distrust of future eventualities and their own ability to deal with potential negative experiences. They fear stepping outside their everyday routines, reluctant to break free from their habitual sphere of action prescribed by cultural tradition and their surrounding institutions. They are unable to let go of their concerns about the uncontrollable consequences of their decisions and actions, and cannot face the inevitable risk with either excited curiosity or a relaxed indifference. They lack the "spirit of play" that proposes decisions in terms such as: "Let's see what happens when, instead of repeating my habitual behaviour, leading me to safe harbour, I take a chance and I head out to a dark and possibly stormy sea." Instead, they keep repeating "but what if … ?" and delay or reject any potentially life-altering decision and the corollary risk. Risk calls for setting oneself against the "what ifs?" and making a decision nevertheless.[5] Insecure people, in moments of indecision, rather than silencing the question with an action, repeatedly turn to their fellow human beings and relate their doubts to them. Søren Kierkegaard, in calling the reader's mind to the stifling effect of endless consultation, voiced this perceptive comparison: "The one whom falling in love does not make silent is not in love, and so also with the true resolution."[6]

In reflections on the relationship between the economic sphere and the play sphere of human life, Huizinga made the following remark: "Pure avarice neither trades, nor plays; it does not gamble. To dare, to take risk, to bear uncertainty, to endure tension – these are the essence of the play spirit."[7] Avarice is an attitude that holds on to the possibilities inherent in one's possessions because of an overwhelming fear of an uncertain future and a lack of confidence in one's capacity to face the consequence of commitment. Just like the person who endlessly only flirts, the miser does not commit himself to the realization of a possibility. He distrusts his capacity to envisage possibilities playfully and take on the risk of investing in one possibility. As Straus asserted, "In every respect the miser reveals himself as a fugitive from the demands of human existence."[8] Those demands consist of acting in the present and creating a present filled with uncertainties and exciting tensions.

The life of the miser, and of all those who refuse to convert potential and abandon certainties, is guided by the need to avoid leaving anything to chance. This fruitless attitude of fear manifests in an absence of elation over a success and a lack of a sense of gratification in what can be a "heightened awareness of I live" (Haigis) in the face of a defeat or a loss. "I have no regrets," wrote Antoine de Saint-Exupéry. "I have played and lost. That is the nature of my profession. At least I have breathed the wind of the sea."[9] These words would never capture the ears of risk-averse people and would never kindle the courage to undertake a daring action – perhaps a hike to a high peak or a persistent questioning of a misleading ideology defended by a political or economical power – for no other reason than to test one's own audacity. We might also mention here the not-uncommon tendency to close the door to a wealth of feelings rather than act in accordance with them, a tendency that leads to the rejection of any all-absorbing commitment.

Doubt about the validity of an impulse and the need to avoid the feeling of anxiety over an uncertain future are not the only reasons for shying away from risks. We might ponder the consequences to others of an unwanted result: to what degree does a risk taken by an individual constitute a risk for a collectivity? In numerous playful or professional activities, another central concern is an evaluation of the timing of a risk. We might, after careful reflection or even an instantaneous assessment of a situation, say that it is not the appropriate time to take the risk or to live with the risk. A given moment in time may not be ripe for giving up the certain for the uncertain.

As I have mentioned above, our reflection involves assessing risk with regard to the form of an activity and the circumstances of its accomplishment. The risk we take by playing tennis is obviously different from the risk we undergo by climbing rock cliffs with no safety gear. Losing a tennis match or suffering a muscle strain affects my mood for a short time. However, if my falling from a certain height leads to a serious injury, the accident deeply affects the life of all those whose well-being depends on me. As we learn about these forms of play, we come to evaluate the risks of our participation. We ask ourselves, is the proposed activity worth the risk? To what degree does this activity, undertaken for pure enjoyment, constitute a risk? The answers to these questions will define our attitude toward a given risk and motivate our decisions in relation to the uncertainties it poses.

These questionings and the ensuing actions can also help a person learn to take risks. This learning takes place first in childhood through various adopted or invented plays, and later, through participation in diverse physical activities. Most children like to be outside – perhaps sledding down a small hill, climbing a tree, or jumping down from a low stone wall. However small the risk of being hurt may seem, these forms of play allow children to acquire the habit of facing uncertainties and going about their play – or any other sort of activity – with an open attitude toward risk.

I venture to think that the attitude one adopts toward risk in childhood remains present in activities carried out later in life beyond the sphere of play, just as the child's curiosity about toys and all sort of things remains alive in the adult's persistent thirst for new knowledge and deeper understanding.

The writer Evelyn Waugh, who travelled extensively to unsafe destinations, declared that risk is indispensable to life itself: "Some measure of physical risk is as necessary to human well-being as physical exercise. I do not mean acts of reckless heroism which are reserved for a minority, and not always the most interesting, of men. But everyone instinctively needs an element of danger and uncertainty in his life."[10] The philosopher Simone Weil held a similar view: "Risk is an essential need of the soul ... In some cases, there is a play (*jeu*) aspect to it; in others, where some definite obligation forces a man to face it, it represents the finest possible stimulant."[11] The desire to take a risk finds its expression in various activities: travelling to a wilderness destination, mountain-climbing, white-water kayaking, freediving in sea caves, and other forms of the so-called risk sports. An apt example is the act of diving into water from a great height, which clearly is not without the risk of hurting oneself. But it also illustrates more subtle aspects of risk-taking. In high-diving, we abandon our habitual and secure position on earth. For a short time, our body experiences a remarkable freedom as it soars through the air, breaks through the frontier between two foreign elements, and with a swoosh reaches into the abyss. The singularity of diving resides in this opportunity to "appropriate" (Sartre), in one continuous action, both elements, air and water, and venture into both directions of our vertical form of spatiality. The firmness of the ground on which we generally stand and walk gives secure support to our movement. When we lift ourselves above the ground and venture into space, we risk falling and suffering an injury. Mountain climbers experience such a feeling during their ascent toward their conquest of a peak. The risk present in diving, however, derives not only from mounting into the void and attaining height but also from leaving our customary upright posture and plunging headfirst into space. Responsible for the feeling of jeopardy is the presence of depth, with all its inherent danger, as well as the peril faced in renouncing our upright posture. Thus, the risk of leaving firm ground is intensely felt while the diver dares to conquer space with the complex movements of spin, twist, and somersault.

At first glance, certain leisure or organized sports activities seem to create occasions for carrying out daring action in "a play spirit," as Huizinga put it.[12] But scholars of sport who emphasize the absence of spontaneity, inventiveness, and improvisation in modern sports would defend another view.

Indeed, studies of numerous characteristics of sport, practised at increasing levels of proficiency, lead them to state that risk is long gone from sport. They forcefully declare that sport is not play and that, even if sport has developed out of the non-utilitarian realm of play and has displayed the spontaneous and imponderable eruption of playful energies, any formal kinship between the two realities no longer exists. These characteristics of modern sports include specialization, rationalization, commercialization, expediency, bureaucracy, and overemphasis of performance, record, and victory. More important, perhaps, is that coaches and athletes tend to view the human body as an object of possession and domination, a performing machine that must be methodically trained with the objective of perfecting its ability to execute a series of complex, standardized, and predictable movements.[13]

Having observed the training of high-level athletes, Christopher Lasch contends that the exaggerated quest for technical perfection and maximal profit has jettisoned the desire to deviate from prescribed routines and take risks, and thus keeps sport apart from the central element of play. "The rationalization of these activities leaves little room for the spirit of arbitrary invention or the disposition to leave things to chance. Risk, daring, and uncertainty – important components of play – have no place in industry or in activities infiltrated by industrial standards, which seek precisely to predict and control the future and to eliminate risk."[14] Lasch seems to be right about the absence of play attitude in many sports competitions, because, as Chesterton so aptly put it, "If you could play unerringly you would not play at all. The moment the game is perfect the game disappears."[15]

Other authors, leaving aside a purely theoretical and ideological motivation, and perhaps because of their concrete and personal involvement in high-level or recreational sports, put forward a more nuanced analysis. Although they separate spontaneous play from rationalized sport and recognize the fundamental differences between these two types of activity, they also contend that the play element and playful reactions do from time to time play a role in sports training and competitions. With this in mind, Schmitz makes the "distinction between forms of play and the spirit which inhabits them," and shrewdly remarks that "This spirit can sometimes animate certain other forms of behavior." Abuses such the desire to win at all cost, the limitless demand for efficiency, and the compulsion to reach financial objectives kill the "spirit of play" in sport and diminish the humanity of players, coaches, managers, and spectators. If these individuals succeed in avoiding such abuses, sport can indeed share certain characteristics with play – "the sense of immediacy, exhilaration, rule-directed behavior, and the indeterminacy of outcome."[16]

In the rationalized and regimented world of sport, we see athletes sporadically discarding their already conceived game plan and expressing their desire to adopt, when the occasion is right, a playful attitude. As they free themselves, even if only briefly, from the imperative of flawless, optimal performance, they may seek and find delight in playfully taken risks: cyclists launch uncalculated early attacks, football players kick "softly-struck chipped penalties," or tennis players make unexpected lobs. Adepts of many disciplines judge on the spot whether a moment is the right time to take a risk, and accomplish their tasks, for a short while at least, with an attitude of play.

In sports, as well as in other forms of standardized activities, we can still see the manifestation of a deep-seated human need to deviate randomly and playfully from prescribed and well-learned forms of movement. I referred earlier to the natural spontaneity of the body, which, by side-stepping any willed determination to repeat what has been learned, effortlessly proposes new ways of moving. Athletes take such unexpected risks either as a result of conscious on-the-spot decisions or in response to a relaxed and trustful surrender to the "intentions" of their "clever body."[17] In rock-climbing or skiing, movement combinations emerge suddenly from the depth of the body; without purposeful pre-assessment or planning, the body creates unusual forms, thereby displaying its own sense of timing and its own judgment of spatial parameters. Alpinists or divers are able to produce surprising and original movements because, as Buytendijk has pointed out, their bodies are invested with "a subtle sense of what can and should be tried, with a *finesse d'esprit*, with an inexhaustible creative power."[18]

I mentioned earlier the act of diving from a height. We might also "dive headlong" into a love relation or into any other enterprise that is imbued with risk and calls for the engagement of our whole being. This kind of diving is seldom accomplished without some preparatory interactions. Every so often, at the very beginning of an encounter between two persons, there is an elusive and magnetic moment during which they feel a sudden but still unclear attraction for each other and discreetly exchange smiles and exploratory glances. How can they break the ice and create the first verbal exchange? Who will take the first step? When is the right time to make the first approach? How will the other person hear the first words? What will the replying voice reveal? With these questions, a playful exchange is set in motion between two persons, an exchange of openness and reticence, a rhythmic oscillation of advance and retreat, marked by the accompanying presence of risk.

If we happen to be part of this experience, we might discover, early in the exchange of glances and words, or after a certain lapse of time, a lack of earnestness in the other person's openness and desire, and notice a sort of alternation between interest and indifference. If so, we are in the presence of someone who is flirting with us. As we have already seen, flirting consists of an unwillingness to bind oneself to a genuine attachment and to surrender to another; it demonstrates a lack of serious-minded commitment; it plays for safety. The interplay of assents and dissents, of allusive promises and withdrawals implies a disinclination to take the risk of being disappointed or wounded. (There is a risk only if one of the partners does not notice this attitude and fails to perceive the other person's non-committal flirtation.)

Georg Simmel, in his analysis of flirtation, defined it as an act of pleasing, of captivating, of accepting to be desired, yet at the same time refusing an affective commitment – in simple terms, playing a game with someone without accepting a risk. Without mentioning it expressly, Simmel's brief and accurate analysis of the flirtatious glance hints at the avoidance of risk. "A sidelong glance with the head half-turned is characteristic of flirtation in its most banal guise."[19] In a casual glance such as this, an inviting attention and a subtle discouragement are simultaneously expressed. The ambivalence of "playful attraction and withdrawal" and the "charm of secrecy and furtiveness" are aptly expressed in a glance that lasts only a second or two. It is only with the elementary directness of a full face-to-face look that a genuine initial liking of the other person and a corresponding uncertainty about the outcome of the encounter come forward.

Simmel's study brings out the distinguishing characteristics of a particular form of human relationship in which a play attitude sustains indecisiveness and ambiguity and simultaneously creates consent and refusal. The true import of his reflections lies, in my opinion, in seeing flirtation as a "ubiquitous experience," not excluding, in principle, any aspect of human life. Simmel points out that flirtation can be seen as a general playful human attitude toward all sorts of realities in our world; one flirts with choices that have few consequences or with decisions about important matters. When we are called to make a decision, we simultaneously, and sometimes even playfully, consider two competing and mutually exclusive possibilities. Since we see the realization of both possibilities as valid and desirable, we keep moving from one to the other, retaining and rejecting each in turn.

This kind of armchair flirting arises out of another fundamental characteristic of human life: indecisiveness. There are issues in our lives in relation to which we are unable take a decisive stand. We then face, for a certain time, possibilities that have equal value and similar appeal. We know that selecting one possibility over another implies a risk and we may be forced to make the painful admission, sometimes only in retrospect, that we failed to make the right decision. Decisions about a profession, a spouse, a place of living, as well as other moral and existential problems, are preceded by the tentative consideration of opposite commitments. Therefore, for a while, before time gives us greater clarity about possible outcomes or reminds us of the urgency of making a decision and taking a risk, we prefer holding both possibilities in our hands and even feel a certain pleasure in this simultaneous "possession." We may also come to the realization that there is sometimes a greater risk in not taking a risk than in living in the disquieting state of uncertainty until the outcome of the selected possibility becomes known.

Let us return to the playful interaction between two persons who turn with genuine interest toward each other. Their glances, smiles, and conversations may be transposed onto a different plane, where the individuals seek more than mere oscillation between affirmation and denial, resistance and deceptive surrender. Here the people involved are entranced in an initial spell that has the potential to grow into a risk-taking attraction.

If flirting involves "concession and withdrawal in the playful rhythm of constant alternation,"[20] the initial exchanges and ensuing conversations between two sensible and sincere individuals nonetheless imply the adoption of a playful attitude of giving and receiving. There is a difference, however, between the glances of a person who flirts and takes a step back and those of a person who merely displays modesty. The former focuses with glacial lucidity on the partner and takes pride in the dissuading effect the last-minute turning-away produces. The latter turns back to him- or herself, fully conscious of the feeling that modesty serves to cover and protect.[21]

In every genuine encounter, there is a reciprocity of openness and holding back, and a harmonious adjustment to what is revealed and what is concealed. This presupposes a desire to create a unity that is simultaneous with an attitude of opposition. Mutual adaptation to what one's partner wants to disclose, as well as reciprocal resistance to an undesirable or early intrusion, sometimes occurs unconsciously according to a tacitly agreed rhythm. Words, gestures, and bodily postures directly convey to a partner the degree of openness or closedness one seeks to achieve at each stage of the encounter. At the same time, one may make adjustments to the degree of one's own openness: self-awareness of this sort allows a person to know when it is the right time to act with little reserve according to a spontaneous impulse and when it is advisable to listen to the voice of reason.

While conversing with each other, partners need to be mindful of the tempo with which they reveal themselves and address personal questions. They need to sense the appropriate approach to the other person by moving back and forth in a playful manner from a trifling observation to a more intimate inquiry. As H.C. Rümke has emphasized in his fine phenomenological study, "In this subtle play of reciprocal opening and closing ourselves, it is precisely the knowledge of the speed adopted by the other which is important."[22] Not being mindful of the right pace is the risk that each partner consciously bears in this play. A hasty self-revelation causes alarm and prompts a definite retreat, and too slow a reaction creates a doubt that deadens the desire to advance further. As in play, it seems advantageous to abandon the will to be in control and thereby to allow the to-and-fro gestures of opening and closing to take place freely, as if by themselves. "Closing and opening ourselves are experiences that happen to us rather than acts that we want expressly to perform."[23] As soon as we attempt to impose our will on this reciprocal playful motion, we risk seeing our partner step back and steer the conversation to safer topics. The place of the encounter, the physical distance between the partners, slight touches of the hands, a change in the inflection of the voices as a new subject is broached – all these and other elements affect the optimal conditions for a gradual mutual opening.

The warmth and receptivity of someone who feels love toward another person is expressed mainly through a direct gaze. Why does the gaze play such a central role in the encounter between two persons who are attracted to each other with a mutual feeling of love? Because the loving gaze goes beyond what constitutes a role or a type and expresses the wish to know the individual traits of the other, his or her genuine personality. Nicolaï Hartmann spoke of a glance (Blick) that does not glide over a face; it "dwells" on it. It rests gently with the other person. Such a "dwelling" requires time, absorption, effort, and not unfrequently a certain daring. The suspicion and ulterior motives that so often guide and define our practical interactions are altogether absent. The recipients of such a loving gaze sense their own worth and dignity and, at the same time, welcome a sincere recognition that can only come from another person. Such recognition acknowledges not merely the bodily appearance but chiefly the unique core of the other person; it sees through what a superficial look would notice and comprehends what makes that person distinct from everyone else.[24]

Still, the risk of failing to create genuine intimacy and a corresponding sense of mutual recognition always remains integral to the playful interaction between two loving persons. Among the literary and operatic testimonials to this risk, perhaps the most famous is Béla Bartók's *Bluebeard's Castle*. As the prologue makes clear, the opera tells a story perhaps recognizable in everyone's life. The dialogue between Judith and Bluebeard expresses the limits to any desire to force a self-revelation too soon and thus to pry into the secret of a soul. It makes its listeners hear and see a portrayal of lack of sensibility with regard to the right timing of a request for greater intimacy. A rigid, over-insistent, and suspicious attitude gradually destroys in the other any inclination to love with greater confidence. To awaken such confidence, one needs to respect the rhythm with which a person's soul reveals itself in order to impart its hopes, riches, and sufferings. As Henri Maldiney has noted, "Friendship and love are made of silent requests in the space already opened by the initial receptivity. It does not use force to reveal a secret. If the other were perfectly transparent, we would go through him and encounter no one."[25]

An adequate treatment of a risk attitude cannot exclude the phenomenon of vertigo. In his book on play, Roger Caillois has crafted a detailed analysis of physical games of vertigo, which generate a pleasurable and frightening intoxication as well as a bodily sensation of disorder and panic.[26] In a subsequent autobiographical book, Caillois pointed out that vertigo is more than a voluntarily induced disruption that can provoke a complete loss of bodily equilibrium; it entails "all sorts of risks and of challenges which imply, in full knowledge, as a probable sanction, the loss of all intellectual, moral, and emotional support, and even of the basis of sheer existence."[27] A capricious or ritualized state of physical disequilibrium and an existential all-pervasive inability to hold on to anything both have their origin in a fundamental human craving to experience the intense panic – the "dreadful rise of emptiness" – that, already in the life of the child, induces both ecstasy and horror. The

writer Fernando Pessoa gave a similar definition of vertigo: "In physical vertigo, there is a whirling of the external world about us; in moral vertigo, of the
interior world. I seemed for a moment to lose the sense of the true relations
of things, to lose comprehension, to fall into an abyss of mental abeyance. It
is a horrible sensation, one that prompts inordinate fear."[28] For Pessoa, this
mental state leads to madness. Caillois speaks rather of a general and compelling need (*un besoin si général et si impérieux*) to take the risk of complete
disorientation offered by the turmoil of human life. He is pleased to have
emphasized forcefully, in his study of play, this neglected basic human need.
"It is a fundamental requirement, a metaphysical one, in a narrow sense of
the term. Something is missing in the life of a human being who has never
felt lost."[29]

In this state of being lost, of having no centre of gravity – no fixed points
of reference – one experiences a profound disruption in the continuity of
one's personal becoming. Just as one's orientation in space is thrown into a
disarray with the dissolution of the stable location from which one is able to
move forward and backward and thus reach one's desired and well-defined
destination, likewise, the perception of lived time undergoes a radical
transformation. The accustomed temporal unfolding of a life path dissipates;
the once-familiar past no longer offers a secure platform for the realization
of possibilities, and future possibilities either recede or seem unreachable.
There is, in the present, no central point where plans and achievements
harmoniously unite, and from which hope and realistic expectation can
motivate further actions.

Such a turmoil and disquieting panic, affecting the very basis of existence,
presents itself when, let us say, someone experiences profound doubts over a
chosen professional vocation. As Louis Lavelle correctly observed, "No one
can wait for the discovery of his calling (*vocation*) before beginning to act:
there comes a moment when he must gamble, and run the risk the gamble
involves."[30] Some individuals playfully consent to the challenge of a vocation and find themselves eventually at a loss, even frightened by the waning
of definite and stimulating directions and points of reference in their lives.
It is worth stressing, once again, that the playful approach to a calling has
nothing to do with careless irresponsibility. When a teacher employed by
a mediocre institution suddenly realizes how debilitating and baneful his
place of work is, the intellectual and emotional confusion about both his past
decision and his future options cuts the ground out from under his feet. He is

thrown back upon himself and seeks to recover his confident, wholehearted, and forward-looking orientation and his initial awareness of the beauty of the chosen vocation or of another quality prompting him to take the risk.

If we return to Caillois's statement that something is missing in the life of a human being who has never felt lost, we might ask what human beings would miss if they had never felt such disarray? I would say that vertigo of an intellectual, moral, or emotional order – the consequence of a gamble over a place, a profession, or a person taken in a playful spirit – makes one feel in his or her bones and sinews the hitherto unimagined polarities of human existence. When one faces the possibility of frightening disorder and a claustrophobic need for a fresh start, one can still attain a singular awareness of being alive. The experience of the abyss brings a captivating reward: an emotional density and breadth are added to an otherwise colourless human life.

I have already touched briefly on the subject of the rise of abstractness and its consequences. The loss of a repeated appreciation of concrete realities leads to a modification in a person's relation to him- or herself. According to Lasch, more and more people bewail a sense of inner impoverishment, emptiness, and coldness – "an inability to feel."[31] They recognize the existence of their bodily self; yet, at the same time, complain about their lack of relation to it; they feel emptiness, "feelinglessness."

When the body is experienced as a distant vacuum or a lifeless reality, the surrounding environment, likewise, appears desolate and arid. Some speak of the waning of the ability to perceive the richness and mobility of their surroundings, of the lack of "feeling of oneness" with the world, and of the severance from the wholeness of things. The possibility of creating a fulfilling relation to people or to things is also deeply disturbed: nothing seems to be concrete or congenial to one's being.

We can now see why people not only participate in rituals and activities that do away with their perceptual and motor sense of stability, but also seek the effects of vertiginous experiences that give them a physical sensation of being alive and a heightened feeling of themselves and the world. Their hopes may be dashed and their life temporarily lack direction, but they are at least able to experience a sense of themselves and consequently to keep an emotional bridge to reality – even if this bridge is, for a certain duration, in ramshackle condition.

6

Humour

"Play," said Émile Buytendijk, "always presupposes a relaxed and un-worried frame of mind that we may call a playful mood (*Stimmung*)."[1] The cheery and light-hearted disposition that leads one to chase after a ball, impersonate a teacher or a neighbour, step into puddles after a rain, or repeatedly jump down from a height is quite natural for healthy children living in security, enjoying the love and liberating support of their parents. Under normal conditions, as we have seen, children respond to the "invitation" of visual or auditory forms and yield to an urge to play. Repeated interaction with these forms often triggers waggish actions, humorous imitations, and whole-hearted laughter. If a child playing on swings with a friend decides jokingly to push his or her partner a bit further than the swing's habitual high point, the recipient of the push, after experiencing a momentary loss of control and a gentle fright, will most likely burst out laughing. They treat their play humorously, and the fun brought into the play enhances their playful mood and sustains the pleasurable continuation of their swinging back and forth.

Admittedly, in certain play activities, the intense concentration required by the task may silence the desire to add humour and create occasions for laughter. Rightly engaged children move their toys with the utmost care and earnestness, and play the role of a pilot or an engineer with a genuine sense of obligation. They go well beyond the simple production of similarities and propose what they conceive as ideal forms of behaviour to be accomplished in an ideal world. They seem to be more thoughtful and to act with more zealous resolve than a hard-working and polite shopkeeper or an attentive and devoted nurse. In their eyes, humour and laughter would offend them and belittle the gravity of their carefully planned and executed activities.

Humour is also absent from games in which the participants practise an activity and take part in competition with assiduous application, discipline, perseverance, and a sense of personal responsibility. All mind games in which the expert participants seek to make the best use of their skills also forbid light-hearted laughter. If we enter a bridge or chess club and observe the behaviour of the players, we see how they exert strict control over their facial expressions and adopt a mask of marmoreal impassivity.

Notwithstanding such notable exceptions, a sense of humour and other forms of play attitude are usually in a relation of reciprocal influence. An unconstrained and responsive mindset generates humorous remarks and imitations, and a humorous outlook prompts a pathic approach to realities. They are often so linked that prioritizing one over the other is hardly possible: a humorous disposition readily suggests a play on enticing words, while a pathic attitude fashions this creativity into humorous caricature of gesture and voice.

A playful attitude, adopted in familiar activities of our everyday lives, often gives prominence to humour. For this reason, Rombach regards humour as a distinct and widely cherished attitude of play: "*Humour* is a playful relation to the world, which can take everything differently and for which everything may also be different."[2] For this difference to exist, things must present themselves under more than one aspect. They are both themselves *and* something else. Humour, then, is the capacity to see and apprehend things in their complexity, ambivalence, and paradoxical nature.

What can playful humour take differently"? What are the other aspects of immediately available realities? Humour brings its contribution to one of the central transformations achieved in play, the manifestation of the potentially expressive and dynamic qualities of things. A humorous disposition allows its possessor to see things and imagine them listening and responding; to see a cloud or a tree and perceive how these realities make grimaces, mimic intentions, present perplexing exaggerations. A child endowed with a sense of humour looks at them with a smile, speaks to them and calls for an answer. In a similar manner, the elementary and immediate objects of the adult world exhibit their expressive presence. Some adults tend to speak in jest to their cars or their devices, especially when these convey an apparent autonomy and fail or delay to respond to their commands. These objects become personalized and are handled as if they were intimate friends; they acquire a distinct significance in their users' lives. Because they seem to take on a life of their own and assert their distinctive characteristics, they are treated and preserved with care and affection. Harold Nicolson's definition applies to this sort of transformation: "Humour is the play of fancy and is content with the comparatively effortless recognition of dissimilarity in similar things."[3] Humour modifies the appearance of the world; it brings life to lifeless reality; it acknowledges the unique and the dissimilar in an otherwise homogenous multiplicity; it sees the dynamic possibilities, novelties, and previously hidden characteristics of things.

Whether introduced knowingly or unknowingly, gradually or suddenly, the imaginative transformation of reality touches on the significance and importance of realities. Humour abstains from any definite valuation of people, their personalities, roles, or actions; it considers them relative and modifiable according to the concrete aspects of a situation. It compares actions and achievements and places them in relation to each other; shifting perspectives make the great appear small and the small great, the impotent omnipotent, the weak powerful. Jokes designed to deflate the stuffy pomposity and vanity of self-satisfied politicians and pretentious scholars are told almost daily. Equally, humour and laughter magnify the aims and realizations of amateur athletic or artistic groups in hopes of ensuring the well-being, cohesion, and conviviality of their members.

Taking everything differently, as Rombach suggests, of course means seeing humour itself under a different light. Just as the above-mentioned cloud or tree is not seen the same way by the farmer, the scientist, the artist, or the child, likewise a humorous perception and reflection can be approached simultaneously from distinct angles – philosophical, aesthetic, sociological, or psychological, for instance. There are diverse points of view on humour, and pretentiously to claim that one is indisputably superior to all others is to suffer both from a lack of a sense of humour itself and from a case of professional deformation. One might study humour as a scientific concept and subject it to a "measurable factor analysis." This approach, as valid and promising as it may be and as many remarkable works as it may have enabled, cannot explain or predict why my chance encounter with an old friend who laughingly tells me an already known joke brings an exquisite and memorable moment to my life. For both the phenomenologist and the psychologist of personality, there remains an elusive aspect to the study of one of the most rewarding and fulfilling of human experiences. Nicolson was persuasive in stating: "our sense of humour is a more intimate, a more confidential, source of amused sensation than our other appreciations of the ludicrous; it occupies a private place in the heart. And whereas our appreciations of wit, satire and irony are always mental appreciations, our sense of humour is a diffused feeling in which sensation and perception are combined."[4] For such reasons, submitting humour to scientific examination and conceptual analysis will hardly yield a comprehensive definition of the personal substance of our sense of humour. We can, to be sure, learn a great deal about humour by examining it in light of the well-known theories, and study the fabric of a particular sense of humour by applying empirical methods. However, even the prominent humorist George Mikes, when perusing this "formidable package" with his discerning eye, did not fail to notice that we still laugh at many things that fall outside of the frame of scholarly inquiry.[5]

There is a latent dialectics of unity and difference in humour inasmuch as it invites us to link a concrete reality with an essence, to apprehend it on an abstract level; conversely, it also asks us to go to life directly, to appreciate an essence in its individual and immediate realization. Such a sense of reality is enacted, for example, when an experience brings us into relation with the body's vulnerability and limitations. The classic misfortune is, of course, the celebrated professor missing the chair and falling down on the floor. We read volumes on the essential qualities of our bodily existence and yet we cannot learn everything about the body's indwelling fallibility or clever intelligence. Humorous incidents and blunders, as well as improvisations and unexpected feats, appear vividly in the performances of actors, musicians, or athletes and give us immediate and unforgettable access both to the body's failures and to its attainments. This is to say that, in the absence of a keen sense of humour, a philosophical approach to human life risks becoming too bookish, divorced from the perception of actual and relevant situations. Rombach goes so far as to suggest the outright prohibition (*Verboten*) of any anthropology that makes no room for laughter and overlooks certain essential and positive dimensions of human experience such as irony, humour, fun, and joke.[6] The anthropology of everyday life will nevertheless fail to make good use of humour and jokes if the philosopher lacks a capacity for surprising and even paradoxical juxtapositions.

We find intimations of this kind of intellectual gift, as well a remarkable sense of humour, in the essays of G.K. Chesterton, who posited that "a joke is always a thought"[7] and that the thought about a man suddenly slipping and falling down on the street is, in truth, chiefly about the "Dual Nature of Man." The act makes immediately manifest "the primary paradox that man is superior to all the things around him and yet at their mercy."[8] It brings to the fore the remarkable human ability to transcend accidents of circumstance, both painful and agreeable ones, as well as the ineluctable obligation to live under all sorts of constraints and dependences. Inevitably, as Chesterton tells us in a regrettably forgotten article published first in the *Encyclopaedia Britannica* and later in a collection of essays, we react initially to a loss of bodily balance with laughter, and our laughter is due to the "purely human realization of the contrast between man's spiritual immensity within and his littleness and restriction without; for it is itself a joke that the home should be larger inside than out."[9] A philosophical reflection may arise from this reaction to a paradox and may draw what Chesterton elsewhere considered a good and useful lesson for a lifetime: "that in everything that matters, the inside is much larger than the outside."[10]

That said, humour may be said to keep alive the philosopher's concern for the concrete dimensions of our existence and to give expression to what Hartmann called the "great need to be true to life."[11] Hartmann put forward the reasons for our recurrent inability to satisfy this requirement. In our everyday lives, as well as in literary works, direct descriptions of the "lower things in life" – all the irritating weaknesses, annoyances, wretchedness, and miseries of our daily existence – risk being too unpleasant and too unbearable for the sensitive person. Humour softens and takes away the rough edges of the body's physical functions; it cancels out, or at least mollifies, the unpleasantness of life's ghastly and distressing realities. Instead of turning our back on our everyday tensions and failures, we are invited to see them from a distance in a liberated state of mind, and enabled to cope with them without feeling their crushing weight.

By its astuteness, humour perceives the discrepancies in human behaviour: it recognizes the gap between appearance and reality; it mistrusts
forms of pompous discourse that traffic in worn-out concepts and empty
phrases, and looks instead for the facts behind the twaddle. Most political
jokes, for instance, debunk the humbug and falsity of the unworthy motives and actions that are all too often linked to oppressive political systems.
Nicolson was in my view wide of the mark in stating that a sense of humour
cannot flourish in a totalitarian society because of the lack of the right balance between convention and exception, acceptance and revolt, conformity
and nonconformity.[12] It seems to me that Mikes, a prolific author of humorous books, has reached a wiser understanding of totalitarian social order and
the vital impact of political jokes on the lives of its citizens. "Under oppressive
regimes jokes replace the press, public debates, parliament and even private
discussion but they are better than any of these. They are better because
serious debate admits two sides, two views; a serious debate puts arguments
which might be considered, turned round, rejected."[13]

There has always been an underground humour adept at exposing the
vices of totalitarian institutions and mentalities, and there always will be. In
addition to the arts, literature, and the vocal or silent resistance of ordinary
courageous persons, humour in its mild or aggressive form keeps people's
sense of things alert. It helps to preserve their sanity and serves as an effective and powerful weapon for challenging and seeing through the deceptive
statements, half-truths, and euphemistic discourses of oppressive and false
regimes, institutions, and cultures. Because humour gives vent to repressed
emotions, subversive humour carries therapeutic value.[14] In times of intimi-
dation and persecution, today just as much as yesterday, the gift of humour
frequently prospers as it nurtures scepticism and doubts about transmitted
ossified norms, rigid bureaucratic procedures, media disinformation, and
misleading abstractions of dominant ideologies and discourses. In the face
of enforced lies, humour seeks to tell the truth. It highlights, above all, the
mismatch between the abstract and the concrete, empty and isolating rhetoric and the experience of the whole of reality, from which genuine thinking
and critical questioning may begin. Humour's sceptical criticism is essential
for locking horns with oppressive powers that are overtly or tacitly present in
workplaces, educational institutions, and cultural communities. Admittedly,
such a sceptical and always-questioning outlook sometimes goes too far and

fails to recognize worthy and authentic intentions. It is the price to be paid for the attainment of a critical approach to all aspects of our life-world, above all for a better understanding of the manipulative power of the intentional misuse of language.

There is nothing inherently humorous in the well-known story of a Jewish man going to see the rabbi.[15] What gives the visit its humorous twist is that it steps outside the normal, the habitual, the orderly, the rational. What makes it funny is that the Jewish man complains to the Rabbi that his son wants to be baptized. The humour consists in putting God and the Jewish man on the same level and portraying them both as fathers who are deeply troubled by the dissent of a new generation. It is the shocking incongruity of the contrast with whatever is normally accepted and included in a social and religious order that creates the humorous effect. Humour sees the unusual and the strange, recognizes them as part of human life, and elicits joy for the richness of life in which the *otherwise*, even in its contrasting and stunning manifestations, is included. The philosopher Joachim Ritter describes our relation to this acutely singular, deviant, and usually excluded or marginalized but secretly present dimension of reality as play, and he sees in the attitude of humour the human disposition to accept the radically other and to take pleasure in its playful presence.[16] Inasmuch as disorder and deviation and abnormality are accepted as part of human life, humour is a philosophy and an existential attitude (*Daseinshaltung*). The humorous attitude makes manifest the "limits of reason" and the positive role of playfulness in our lives. By making room for the strange, the alien, and the messy, humour can be included in the creative development of our professional activities and of our real and sometimes chaotic existence.[17]

We sometimes witness the irruption of the abnormal into our life-world. The incursion happens unexpectedly, as when, for example, elated goal-scoring players express their joy with an amusing dance or a frolicsome jumping up and down. Their ardent supporters take perhaps just as much delight in these frequent and inventive moments of celebration as in the players' athletic prowess. Leaving behind the seriousness of rivalry, the players also enjoy their act of initiating a spontaneous farce with light-hearted playfulness. For a few precious seconds, the exuberance of the hilarious and disorderly dance or antics takes over from controlled and orderly performance. In many other such communal situations – a solemn graduation ceremony, for instance – participants may find amusement in suddenly disrupting an orderly event.

They may react with unexpected and unbridled movements of their bodies in response to the recognition bestowed upon them.

Israel Knox presented an inadequate view of sports activities when he stated that the element of humorous playfulness had by the 1950s "almost totally vanished" from baseball and American football. He was right, however, in describing humour as the irruption of "playful chaos in a serious world," and claiming that "the very playfulness of its chaos suggests that it does not disown the world, [but] that it grants its lovers the boon of a holiday."[18]

The disruptive and contrasting nature of humour and the inclusion of the strange, quirky, and uncommon in our lives are immediately and distinctly apparent in practical jokes. These create unexpected situations and a certain deformation of the realities that normally guide and influence our actions. Practical jokes are intended to deceive their selected victims and to create in them, for a time at least, a degree of perplexity, confusion, and embarrassment. They call for the creative invention of a mischievous act, a sort of trap, and its skilful insertion into the normal course of events, resulting in the transformation of a situation, the disarray of the victim, and the contentment of the joker. There is pleasure in planning the joke ahead of time and toying with various imagined forms of execution. And there is malicious enjoyment in observing the victim's falling for the prank and subsequently learning the truth. "The satisfaction of the practical joker," observed W.H. Auden, "is the look of astonishment on the faces of others when they learn that all the time they were convinced that they were thinking and acting on their own initiative, they were actually the puppets of another's will."[19]

Aggressive and nasty jokes seek to deflate pride, to demolish conceit, or to achieve vicious aims with implicit or explicit cruelty. Mild jokes are designed and carried out with an impish yet sympathetic mindset; their authors seek to generate momentary puzzlement, disorientation, and uncertainty rather than sordid humiliation or personal injury. The philosopher Michel Serres has expressed his love of such rowdy acts, which are absurd, illogical, and harmless. In his book entitled *Morales espiègles* (Mischievous Morals), he has recounted with "gentle laughter" the model of the ideal practical joke.

This joke was devised and perpetrated by two students of the École normale supérieure – Serres admiringly labelled them "princes of mischief" – on the arrival of a foreign dignitary. They stole a giraffe from Paris's *Jardin des plantes*, brought it to the airport in a van with a sliding roof, and skilfully merged their vehicle behind the presidential convoy. After their arrival at the *Elysée*, they presented the giraffe to the master of ceremonies as the gift of the foreign guest to the host, General de Gaulle. Then, the master of ceremonies asked the general to thank the distinguished visitor who, of course, knew nothing about his own "generous gift" and who had never even seen a giraffe in his own country. Meanwhile, the giraffe, with its impressive stature, had wreaked havoc in the unfamiliar environment. Hearing and seeing the disruption caused by the restless animal, the general instructed his prime minister, Georges Pompidou, to put an end to the *fracas*. When the unruly long-necked ruminant was taken away and the identity of the irreverently laughing comrades was learned, the furious and forthright Pompidou threatened them with imprisonment. Serres, for his part, thought that, in recognition of their puckish inventiveness, they deserved rather the *Légion d'honneur.*[20]

Practical jokes consist essentially of creating an unusual and awkward situation that baffles the victims and pushes them "out of time." Henri Bergson was surely perceptive to claim, in his widely read book *Le rire*, that everyday life calls for adaptation to expected situations rather than distraction.[21] Habitual actions linked to already-known situations ensure the confident undertaking of tasks designed for the orderly attainment of objectives in the future. Practical jokes have the aim of interrupting the normal sequence of events; their befuddled victims are deflected from their anticipated seamless and adaptive progress to the future. To the victim of a practical joke, the present is no longer lived as a solid and broad ground supporting the realization of previously envisaged tasks. The victims hurriedly turn to the future in search of a saving solution. By creating an entirely novel situation, the deviser of an unexpected joke plays with time: the joke is meant to produce a collapse of the habitual continuity of time.

I was going to write "helpless and defenceless victims." But an elegant joke designed without malice or hatred always gives its intended victims a slight chance to find ways of freeing themselves from the trap. If they can succeed in coming up with a suitable response quickly and efficiently, their clever way of parrying the consequence of a well-designed mischief may become in itself a good cause for laughter. The jokesters know the possible implications of the novel situation and can therefore see it from both points of view, that of the victim and their own. This knowledge and the victim's obligation to deal with the situation provide the practical joker with a certain power over the victim's immediate destiny and arouse the pleasure of being able to influence, to a certain extent, the victim's feelings and actions. But there is more. While fooling others, the michief-makers are equally exposed to being fooled in their turn. Elfish jokers expect to become eventual victims themselves and, if they have a genuine sense of humour, find great fun in the experience of reciprocity. Thus, the playfulness of these acts is enhanced by the victims' inclination to retaliate and, at a favourable moment, to devise a new joke against those who initially sought to embarrass them. Their riposte will most likely be followed by another retaliation, and this back-and-forth leg-pulling can go on as long as the participants are inventive, have a similar sense of humour, and are fond of braving jokes.

It may happen, however, as Ludwig Wittgenstein has observed, that two persons do not have the same sense of humour. "They do not react properly to each other."[22] Wittgenstein has compared this mismatch to a situation in which one person throws a ball to another, who, instead of throwing it back, puts it into his pocket. I should note about this pertinent comparison that an outsider would most likely perceive the contrast between the two forms of behaviour as amusing. As simple as this scene may appear to an outside observer, seeing it as laughable nevertheless requires the contribution of intelligence. For one of the achievements of the human intelligence is the simultaneous apprehension of opposing contraries.[23]

Our intelligence perceives or introduces one of the central elements of humour: an incongruity between two realities that, for some reason, do not fit "properly with each other." On all levels of our daily lives we find recurring incongruities between idea and fact, the expected and the actual, order and disorder, sense and nonsense, normal and abnormal, the lifeless and the living – or, as Chesterton emphasized, the inside and the outside. When we make a funny remark or tell a joke, we shrewdly juxtapose two usually incompatible realities, statements, codes of behaviour, points of view, or contexts.[24]

One might affirm that seeing an event as humorous depends not solely on one's sense of the incongruous but also, and primarily, on the circumstances pertaining to the life-world in which the event occurs. These circumstances, including language, cultural tradition, social convention, and individual disposition, determine what an onlooker singles out as laughable in an event. Linking someone's sense of humour to social conditions may provide plausible reasons for Wittgenstein's observation. Admittedly, a joke invented and told with glee in Japan can easily fall flat in France, while a scene on a

Parisian boulevard, which a French host views as completely comic, would appear egregious and irreverent to a Japanese tourist. I would argue, however, that watching a soccer player lose his shorts during a match is likely to provoke the same hilarity everywhere around the globe. The incongruity of a naked buttock still running after a ball during a strenuous athletic contest transcends spatial and temporal relativities. In many instances, humour can produce the same atmosphere of common understanding and conviviality among strangers as music and dance, which are also forms of play. Martha Nussbaum has seized on this point: "The forms that play takes are enormously varied; yet we recognize other humans, across cultural barriers, as the animals who laugh. Laughter and play are frequently among the deepest and also the first modes of our mutual recognition."[25] Mutual recognition presupposes a mutual understanding of the reasons behind laughter and play. To understand a funny story or scene is to be able to identify its elements, bring them together, and see the impact created by their interrelation. Beyond the great number of jokes presenting specific actions and characteristics, and calling for a national or topical sense of humour, are an even greater number of droll actions and comical events that occur at airports, public squares, conferences, or athletic competitions and instantaneously help overcome barriers of separateness by fostering a laughing community of humour.

How does a playful, humorous attitude manifest during interactions with our fellow human beings or in the presence of tasks that we are called to accomplish? As we saw earlier, cheerfulness is one of the fundamental moods that generate humorous observations and practical jokes. Cheerful individuals display a remarkable ability to see themselves and their situation in a mirthful and light-hearted manner, as it were from an alternative viewpoint, and at the same time to rise above the constraining and even oppressive power of external influences.[26]

Those who have written about the innumerable tragedies experienced under totalitarian regimes have repeatedly come to the same question: how could such people survive imprisonment, deportation, and the period that followed with a strong spirit and dignity? There seems to be a consensus that, beyond the help of relatives and friends, their faith, sense of self-worth, strong desire to live, and sense of humour were what helped the most.

With humour, a serious and even tragic reality is coupled with the ability to place this reality in a framework in which, for a certain time at least, its gravity is suspended or accepted as tolerable. Humour takes note of all the painful adversities arising in hostile circumstances and, through the adoption of an attitude of detachment, looks beyond them and gives assent to existence. It achieves this by dispelling the desire to entertain self-deceiving illusions and nurturing, rather, the sense of ordinary and simple things in life such as a conversation with a friend or the joy of feeling the warmth of the sun while sitting on a bench in a park. It is in moments of hardship that humour comes to the rescue of humans and incites them to crack a life-enhancing joke. Leroi-Gourhan, thinking about this saving force of humour, declared, "In its absence, we would become the miserable creatures that we can too easily imagine."[27]

Paradoxically, we have to treat some of our serious concerns with unfettered detachment if we are to approach human life with utmost earnestness. Such a disposition to recognize and live with the polarities of existence has its source in humour; as Frederick Neumann points out, "The essence of humorous logic consists of suddenly imputing to humans their own opposites."[28] I would add to this observation that the essence of playfulness consists in illuminating and revealing, by contrast and from a distance, the existential inconsequence of what we hold to be so vital and so serious in our lives. We do not cease to value earnestness; for a time, we merely attach it to another object or occupation. We are able to undergo hardship and persist in clinging to our most earnest concerns because, at the same time, we are also able to treat them light-heartedly and with detachment. The political dissident Vaclav Havel maintained that individuals living and working under irksome totalitarian constrictions were able to realize their serious political and artistic objectives thanks only to the preservation of a sense of humour and an attitude of derision. Losing the easy gaiety of humour implies losing the earnest quality of an activity. As Havel wrote, "An act can become important provided that it is accomplished by a man who is aware of the temporal and futile nature of all that is human."[29] Humour provides insight into the possible disproportion between investment and result. Curiously enough, noting the eventual disparity with a smile serves to enhance one's devotion to a cherished cause.

The validity of this approach upheld by Havel can be verified in numerous occupations of our lives. Taking things too seriously, with a rigid, pedantic, inflexible approach, often leads to failure – sometimes even to catastrophic results. One of the shortcomings of overly serious persons is the inability to accept the absurdity of their actions; they tend to deny that many of their conscientious and strenuous efforts may lead, after all, nowhere and prove to be pointless. A sense of humour provides us with the indispensable detachment and elasticity to live with the absurd and let go with alacrity and no bitterness. This is a precious and vital aspect of the capacity for humour. And because in the spirit of humour we can envisage the experience of the absurd and even become its advocate, we are able to pursue our valued activities with the utmost passion. We have this capacity because, to borrow the words of Ludwig Radermacher, we understand "existence in terms of contradictions and deal with the earnest by means of its opposite."[30]

The closeness and interdependence of earnest and light-hearted attitudes has received brilliant treatment in Hugo Rahner's book on play.[31] Rahner proposes a Christian interpretation of the humanistic ideal of the "grave-merry" man, which had been analyzed at length by E.R. Curtius.[32] Bringing jollity and gravity into unity and balance, this Christian ideal of former times may also be adopted in the bustle of our own everyday lives. It represents a way of accomplishing such practical activities as meeting a business partner, delivering a weekly report to a smaller group, repairing a house, or taking on other habitual tasks by alternating or combining serious and lighter approaches. In striving to live up to this ideal, we are aware of all sorts of obligations and duties that require application and perseverance, and yet we are also able to carry them out with a jaunty and humorous predisposition. We strive to cope with life's tasks and challenges as well as possible and accept all shortcomings, disappointments, and failings – our own and those of others. We do not cancel out the multiple constrictions imposed by our social environments and private milieus; lightness of playful humour grants us a temporary relief from the burden and stress of life and offers occasions for regaining some of the energies consumed by life's routine cares.

When we say that grave-merry persons have a humorous outlook on their public and private lives, we also understand this stance particularly in relation to the obligation of making decisions; this attitude accepts with equanimity the inherent solitude, the discarded possibilities, and the possible sombre consequences of any decision. Decisions are among life's greatest challenges, especially when alternative possibilities exert comparable appeal and when the voice of reason and the prompting of the heart press upon the hesitating person with equal persuasive force. Humour nurtures a more carefree approach toward what seems at first to be a "monumental concern." It knows and accepts that whichever – the heart or the reason – emerges as more persuasive, the outcome remains uncertain, and may cause inevitable disappointment.[33]

Mikes has written on humour with intelligence and sympathy, treating it as one of the "greatest gifts of humanity."[34] His fondness for the subject did not stop him from declaring that humour is essentially "cruel and aggressive" and that not all those who have a sense of humour are amiable individuals. In his book on the death of humour (the content of which proves rather that, in some circles, humour is alive and more vigorous than ever before), Mikes asserts unequivocally: "Humour is always aggressive, hostile, and often cruel."[35] Even the mildest jokes, he says, may convey a strong attack on an established social or political order or on individuals' unbending habits and outdated conventions. By keeping alive the sense of truth, caustic humour fosters and sustains a vigorous opposition to oppressive ideologies and a sharp criticism of false claims to personal glory. According to Mikes, hostility and cruelty find their outlet chiefly in practical jokes and wry witticisms, which, by dint of their irresistible repetition, have become a way of life in some artistic and literary circles.

Chesterton brought a more nuanced approach to the use of the terms. Wit, he stated, is the intellect's judgment projected onto others, and humour is by turns the subtle or brazen way of commenting on the humorist's life and action. Wit seeks an advantage over other persons by singling out their shortcomings quickly and deliberately, and by suggesting corrective measures. Humour is calmer and more peaceful; it observes with sympathy and objectivity how these same persons behave in their concrete environment, what desires they have, what actions they undertake, and what results they achieve; should it bump up against human frailties, it treats them with understanding and no desire to correct or reject them. The receptivity of humour, as Chesterton suggested, goes together with an honest sideways look at oneself and, if any scolding is to be done, it begins with oneself. "Humour always has in it some idea of the humourist himself being at a disadvantage and caught in the entanglements and contradictions of human life."[36] Therefore, "wit corresponds to the divine virtue of justice," and humour to "the human virtue of humility."[37] Humour presupposes the ability to see oneself with a sense of proportion, to recognize one's weakness, vanity, errors, foibles, and silliness, and to laugh at them unreservedly.

We can see that there are at least two fundamentally different ways of outlining the condition of humour: one might claim that humour comes from dispositions of sympathy, kindness, and friendliness, while another might think that it is fuelled by feelings of antipathy, cruelty, and hostility. The humorist can thus be seen either as a gentle and likable soul or as an aggressive and destructive creature hiding behind a charming smile. We have here more than simply two philosophical interpretations of the mental origins of humour. Enmity and affability, as well as other possible qualities such as jealousy, conceit, heartlessness, compassion, solidarity, and joviality are all general and consistent modes of seeing things. They and their opposites assert themselves as conscious or subconscious habits functioning in all sorts of circumstances of everyday life. They leave their mark on a person's sense of humour and on the sense of wit and the other (ironical, satirical, sarcastic) ways of relating to life's incongruities and other whimsical moments. "Humour," alleged Hartmann, "is an affair of an ethos, conditioned by character and reflecting one's entire picture of life; this ethos stands behind one's sense of humour, and probably that sense was first provoked by the ethos. In any case, the ethos is what gives it the characteristic coloration of one's benevolence and good humour."[38] For Hartmann, contrary to Mikes, the *ethos* that motivates and defines the formal aspects of a humorous remark or observation about a comical reality is warm-hearted and sympathetic. This reality might be altogether silly. Yet a person who notices the asinine incongruity of a situation is not satisfied with a superficial approach; he or she reaches to a deeper level and uncovers appealing and amiable traits in a person's the seemingly foolish and fatuous behaviour.[39] Hartmann spoke of the "ethos of laughter" which reveals a person's "entire attitude towards life (*eine ganze Lebenshaltung*)." We need only observe how people laugh to detect, in their bodily expression, the distinct quality of their attitudes toward the object of their laughter as well as toward all the other aspects of their lives. There are, of course, as many sorts of laughter as there are ways of seeing the comical in a given situation or as there are ways of being and acting in the world. Wit, sarcasm, irony, satire, jest, derision, and humour are among the possible ways of apprehending, and responding to, the comic or incongruous. Each of these responses springs from an individual's way of thinking, feeling, and acting. A group of persons will probably react in a similar manner to a perceived hilarious event. Even so, unanimous laughter still presupposes an individual perception of the event and the possibility of not joining in the collective uproar.

I am inclined to share the views of Hartmann, Chesterton, and others who have asserted that the *ethos* of humour is receptive, peaceful, conciliatory, and broadminded. To my mind, Mikes and his spiritual father, Martin Grotjahn, are mistaken even if it is not always possible to detect a humorist's true intention in a joke. Numerous publications on styles of humour and the personality traits of the humorist give diverse explanations on this issue.[40] In such situations, philosophers are advised to rely on their own experiences in formulating their ideas on inductive grounds, and to accept, with a conciliatory and unswerving sense of humour, a disagreement about the foundation of their own sense of incongruity. They might share, as I do, the conclusion of Nicolson, who studied the topic with a "wholly objective attitude": "It [humour] may not be the index of a very active intellect, but it is certainly the index of a most agreeable temperament."[41] Hartmann agreed with this perspective: "The eye of the humourist is fundamentally full of love and sympathy; he even shows favour to the human weaknesses he reveals."[42]

Of course, we are not always able to see a person or an action with a feeling of love or sympathy. But we are at least able to put up with others' views and actions and treat them with a smile or a shrug of our shoulders. By doing so, we take a distance from our ingrained ideas, established habits, and cherished purposes and view them as if from a superior point of view. This distance also secures a certain protection from all sorts of tensions and predicaments that we might otherwise apprehend and carry within us; it minimizes their power. Humour offers, then, a form of transcendence that allows us to disengage ourselves, at least for a short time, from all sorts of disagreeable and uncomfortable situations. In the midst of our staid tasks, we find genuine repose in humour. Anyone who has felt the fatigue brought on by concentration on the content of a lecture or any sort of presentation can appreciate the soothing detachment provided by a humorous remark. The steadying influence of humour is felt in the most diverse circumstances: during a stressful job interview, before a decisive athletic competition, or after a winsome woman or man impassively repelled one's courteous and proper advances.

I have already stated that humorous remarks or imitations, advanced with a playful attitude, and their ensuing laughter can bring two persons together even if they come from different cultures and their encounter is ephemeral. Roger Scruton caught well that mood when he remarked that, while telling jokes to each other or laughing together at a comedy, we establish and create a friendlier relation to our fellow human beings: "in all its forms laughter is a social response: more, it is a *society-building* response."[43] Even more so,

I would add, it triggers a tolerance-building response. In a book first issued during the "Great War" with an underlying hope of creating a less belliger-ent world, Richard King stressed the magnetic power of humour: "A mutual sense of humour is more binding than a mutual ideal. People who have once had a good laugh together can never afterwards be real enemies."[44] Two quar-relling neighbours, or two disagreeing and even hostile university professors who succeed in smoothing the way for a rapprochement confirm the validity of this observation. Given the opportunity to spend an hour or two together, share a meal and a bottle of wine, crack a few jokes, and laugh heartily, they are more likely able to put up with their differences, make conciliatory ges-tures, and cease to maintain their feud and its associated huffy and vengeful feelings. And persons who have been raised in dissimilar environments and traditions would better understand each other if each of them made an effort to learn about the sense of humour of a foreign ethnic group.[45]

What makes the engine of a car or any similar kind of machine run well? When the bolts and gears are not tightened too much and when they are al-lowed a little play. And, of course, when oil reduces the friction of the moving parts. Similarly, the social machine runs well when a certain play within its parts is allowed and a lubricating substance is provided. Humour and laugh-ter furnish the "engine of the society" with the necessary play and with the indispensable lubricant oil. Instantaneously, humour makes conversing peo-ple relaxed and casual. While laughing, they no longer maintain their stiff upright posture and even forgo control over their body. The loss of strict composure in their stance makes them more receptive to each other. No lon-ger are they overly cautious partners who are on guard, keep their faces and hands immobile, and measure their words with care. If they laugh together, they are more likely to reach a common understanding and come to an ini-tial agreement about something in the world. They reveal something about themselves and perhaps even disclose shortcomings as well as the manner by which they may come to terms with them. Humour is often indifferent to rigorous cultural, economic, and professional distinctions; it allows all mem-bers of a society to find common ground and to share concerns and burdens without bitterness or resentment. A community that can spontaneously and laughingly find a way to talk about both its lamentable imperfections and its corrective aspirations will, as Scruton proposes, end up "viewing life with cheerful equanimity" and with healthy common sense.[46]

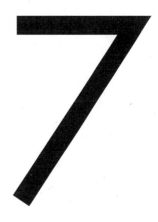

Gratuité

I n his article on play mentioned earlier, Émile Benveniste made an observation pregnant with meaning: "In all ages, whether one lets it happen or looks for it, playing means forgetting the useful, beneficially submitting oneself to the forces that real-life conditions curb and harm."[1] In our everyday lives, we turn to the useful, interact with it, and shape our activities according to its limiting constraints and enabling possibilities. The principle of usefulness runs through many of our habitual actions and interactions, whether they are carried out at home, at work, or while travelling or otherwise enlarging our stock of knowledge. Taking a bus and buying food are useful pursuits in relation to desired ends. Nevertheless, while we travel to our workplace or run some errands, we do not think explicitly about the usefulness of our means of transportation or the purchased objects. We forget the useful, partly because our goal is our central concern, partly because the useful has become as familiar as the air we breathe or as habitual as our automatically accomplished movements. Usefulness determines the quality of the overall atmosphere within our everyday existence; this atmosphere leaves its mark on human actions and interactions, perception of things and their contexts, experience of space and time; and at the same time, because of its closeness and familiarity, it escapes our explicit awareness. We detect it when something goes wrong, our bus is late, our car does not start, or our employer encounters financial difficulties and our colleague comes to work in a gloomy mood.

Benveniste does not have this sort of forgetfulness in mind. Forgetting the useful means, for him, leaving behind instrumental and utilitarian concerns and entering a domain in which realities and objectives are seen in a different light and behaviour undertaken in relation to these objectives is modified accordingly. In play, activities and things are valued independently of their possible or real usefulness; they are not regarded or handled as means to attain some desired ends.

This quality of explicit uselessness, or gratuitousness, has been repeatedly emphasized in studies on play. Inspired by the publications of the Swiss biologist Adolf Portmann on the "world of living beings" and the "incredible richness of living forms," Buytendijk has brought forward the purpose-free character of human play in relation to all the useless and "functionless" forms and behaviour that are on display in the natural world.[2] He has written of the "playful abundance of the organic nature" that we are able to apprehend intuitively. This wealth is present in the guise of the "self-representation" and "self-formation" of countless living beings, and contrasts with all the purposeful structures and functions that are indispensable for their self-preservation. We find the display of the same sort of "playful abundance of forms" in our human existence; admittedly, it is transposed to, and lived out upon, another level, but is nevertheless quite different from life's necessities and strictly useful elements. "The human being is not only a *homo faber* but also a *homo ludens* … The human being is a *player*, because he is a *homo sapiens* and because *sapientia* exhibits an original relationship to *sapere*, to tasting, to taste."[3] Taste is understood here as an intimate sensory perception and a refined enjoyment of what is beyond the utilitarian. Whereas the useful is often valued collectively, the object of our taste is cherished individually, even if a person enjoys something in company of others.

Some years before Buytendijk wrote about the "idea of the purposeless profusion of living forms," Romano Guardini advanced perceptive distinctions in his books on liturgy and works of art.[4] He presented two principles or standpoints that determine how things are seen and valued and how actions are learned and accomplished. According to the principle of purpose (*Zweck*), actions and objects are useful means to attain certain ends. Realities are considered in relation to their purpose, and their value is assessed according to the criteria of usefulness. Guardini, who in his books combines wide reading with knowledge of the world, was surely right in observing that, although appropriate and necessary for the achievement of social, economical, and technological objectives, the standpoint of purpose, coupled with instrumental reasoning, is insufficient to our understanding and valuation of all dimensions of human life. We encounter things and witness events that are neither intended nor deemed purposeful; they nevertheless present themselves with an intrinsic meaning (*Sinn*). "This meaning is not realized by their extraneous effect or by the contribution which they make to the stability or the modification of another object, but their significance consists in being what they are. Measured by the strict sense of the word, they are purposeless, but still full of meaning."[5] Play must be viewed from the standpoint of meaning; it is activity that has no other aim than to produce "purposeless actions" spontaneously and in an orderly manner. Useless play, then, provides enjoyment to all participants as long as no educational intentions or methods overburden and falsify it.

Two seemingly contradictory but, in reality, complementary characteristics are exhibited and shared by play and liturgy. In both activities, movements are executed according to "gravely drawn up rules," while the objects are handled with utmost care and respect. Yet, at the same time, both play and liturgy allow the participants to produce an abundance of words, movements, and actions without measuring or justifying them by the objective standard of strict suitability for a purpose. What Guardini said about play applies as well to the ritual of liturgy: "it is life, pouring itself forth without an aim, seizing upon riches from its own abundant store, significant through the fact of its existence."[6]

Guardini has reflected on a range of activities – professional, scientific, legislative, artistic, ecclesiastical, and liturgical – in relation to purpose and of meaning. He has also succinctly described the motives that guide the child who plays and inspire the artist who creates. In so doing, he has highlighted two forms of attitude: "state of mind" (*Seelenzustand*) and "inclination" (*Geistesart*), or simply "spirit" (*Geist*) – as in "pragmatic spirit" (*Geist der Sachlichkeit*) – which become manifest in all walks of human life. The concepts that most successfully capture the central elements of each of these attitudes are *usefulness* and *uselessness*. The French equivalents, *utilité* and *gratuité*, perhaps provide a more elegant expression of this polarity.[7]

As we have seen in the previous chapters, the attitude adopted and nurtured in play animates and shapes countless human endeavours. How does the attitude of *gratuité*, central to all play, become apparent in our overt actions? I should like to think that a tangible experience, shared by many readers, tells us more about the idea of *gratuité* than any dry and abstract theory. Consequently, I discuss here two forms of activity that are enjoyed for their intrinsic worth, drinking wine and strolling, well knowing that numerous other kinds of concrete pursuits are equally deserving of mention and could just as well illustrate this principle of a playful way of acting and living.

Drinking wine seems to be a common and shared way of shaping one's action with an attitude of *gratuité*. I approach this topic with the help of Béla Hamvas, who addressed the subject playfully and earnestly in his book *The Philosophy of Wine*. It is perhaps not a philosophical treatise from the point of view of contemporary analytical thinkers. It is, rather, a good-humoured and thought-provoking book, short and enjoyable to read. Since it is a serious reflection on, and deft guide to, a certain way of life, the book's title is not unjustified. Serious, of course, does not mean hermetic or boring. I would compare Hamvas's reflections to Joseph Haydn's symphonies; these are full of original and carefully constructed musical ideas and, at the same time, witty, captivating, and fun to listen to.

In the spring of 1945, after the capture of Budapest by the Red Army, Hamvas returned to his home. His house had been bombed. He had lost everything he owned, cherished, and had created; his manuscripts, books, and furniture had all been destroyed. A few weeks later, he travelled to Hungary's Lake Balaton and wrote a series of remarkable meditations on wine. These thoughts eventually became one of his most beautiful, liberating, and successful books. Many years later, Roger Scruton, in his philosopher's guide to wine and meditation on drinking, paid a short tribute to Hamvas and expressed the hope, not without an added touch of dry humour, that Hamvas's book would never be translated into English.[8]

To be sure, Hamvas writes about vineyards and wines. He views wines as if they were living beings, each displaying a definite personality and acting of its own accord. Although sketchy and incomplete, his catalogue of wines is a remarkable phenomenological achievement; just as the playing child sees animated realities in all the surrounding objects, likewise Hamvas recognizes in the wines he tastes numerous characteristic qualities such as charming smiles, good manners, laziness, undemanding sense of humour, heroic passion, faithfulness, silence, and calm. Wine drinking, if it occurs under suitable conditions, is a life-enhancing experience. It can give us a previously unknown sense of peace and serenity. Gazing at the wine's colour for a minute or two, relishing its aromatic characteristics, savouring its particular flavour, all while seated near the entrance of the cellar, under a nut tree, with a view on the parallel rows of vines in the vineyard, are acts that create an undefinable and profound affective resonance in us. Each has its singular and personal value, which calls for no extrinsic justification and eludes any attempt to capture it in words. We are in intimate union with the wine and the cultivated landscape of viticulture, and we take a heightened pleasure in this feeling of harmony and equivalence.

Regulating this kind of experience by strict laws, writes Hamvas, is therefore both misguided and unhealthy. Laws breed hypocrisy, pedantry, calculation, and, above all, unhappiness. With regard to drinking, we must answer to one law alone: anywhere, anytime, anyhow. Still, "we must awake in us the instinct that gives drinking dignity."[9] What can we say about this instinct for dignity? Since each wine has a distinct personality, we must carefully choose the appropriate food, place, time, and even glass for the wine we intend to drink. The characteristic of the wine should determine even the number of persons tasting and enjoying it; there are wines for persons drinking alone and wines that should be enjoyed only in a small group. The latter call for music and do not endure solitude. As in other carefree activities, the circumstances are of the highest importance. There are wines to be served only in taverns. Hamvas considers the tavern a vital institution of our civilization, much more important than, for instance, the parliament. In the latter, wounds are inflicted; in the former, they are healed.[10] The sensibility for wine drinking is, in fact, evident nowhere more than in the care taken in the formality, the ceremony, even the ritual. Scruton wholeheartedly agrees on this point: "Drinking precious wine is preceded by an elaborate process of separation, which has much in common with the ablutions that preceded ancient religious sacrifices. The bottle is retrieved from some secret place where the gods have guarded it; it is brought reverentially to the table, dusted off and uncorked with a slow and graceful movement while the guests watch in awed silence ... The wine must then be swirled, sniffed and commented upon, and only when all this is duly accomplished can it be poured with ceremonial priestcraft into the glasses."[11]

Drinking while in such a right frame of mind has nothing to do with wild debauchery or the unrestrained expression of impulses. Beyond the pleasure of tasting the wine and beyond the joy of feeling "the root of every intoxication, love,"[12] drinking at a social gathering is an invitation to chatter, sing, dance, make merry, and, above all, to perceive and enjoy tangible realities. It is an occasion to view wine as if through the eyes of a poet or a playing child who sees in it those expressive and dynamic qualities that animate it and give it life. The French sociologist Pierre Sansot also stressed this intimate relation between wine drinking and poetry: "If poetry has the capacity to reveal one aspect of Being, if it is sometimes born from a subtle, discreet, moving harmony between persons, places, and seasons, we must admit that the ordinary consumption of wine is poetical."[13] Drinking wine in everyday or festive circumstances invites us to become familiar with a rhythmic combination of vivid forms without any concern for their usefulness. (Even winemakers and wine merchants are able to adopt, occasionally, such an attitude. They may enjoy the wine, the spirit of a cellar, the conversation with viticulture workers without thinking about the monetary benefits from the sales.) Such an attitude – one that we might adopt in the presence of a colourful prairie landscape or a Schubert sonata – presupposes a freedom from all the limitations imposed by a purely utilitarian understanding of the world. If we prepare the table with particular care, carry out the slow ceremony of the cork, taste the wine with gentle sips, and amicably and freely converse about the latest sports events or burning metaphysical questions, or read aloud from a book of poetry, we tend to emphasize the intrinsic value of the moment.

There is another playful activity that Hamvas barely mentions but which goes well with civilized drinking among friends: group-singing. Unless obtrusive and irritating background music drowns them out, songs may be heartily performed by a group of people seated around a table on benches, glass in hand, in a state of light intoxication. Drinking songs are not forms of celebration of the quality and hallmarks of particular wines or of successful grape harvesting. They are, rather, humorous ways of expressing the high spirits produced by the wine, accompanied sometimes by a command to drain the glass during the final sustained tonic note. A person alone drinks, happily or sadly, in silence. But a group of friends or strangers brought spontaneously together add to the delight of drinking all the colours of the singing voice and the atmospheric quality created by the song. Repetition of the melody and variations on the words give these songs at times a joyful and jesting character, at times a melancholic and nostalgic tone. A "community of consonance" (Straus) is formed when people come together and enjoy the heady effect of the sounds produced perhaps even more than the flavour of the wine savoured; the singing creates a genuine sense of belonging.

Relishing wine gives us sensory pleasure: we observe the wine's colour, inhale its bouquet, taste its qualities. Our visual and olfactory senses also absorb the circumstances of our gustatory experience: the glasses, the bottles, the table cloth, the room, the cellar, or the garden. We are exposed to various aromas and with them to the affective qualities of an overall atmosphere. If the aroma produces in us an agreeable sensation, we feel ourselves in synchrony with the prevailing atmosphere. Discerning a pleasant aroma is more than a sensory experience; it is the foundation of our pathic attitude of opening ourselves to an ambience in which we are gently seized by an affective quality and feel at ease and at home. Similarly, tasting is more than a mode of sensory contact of the tongue and the palate with an object. While tasting the charm of a village tavern or the harmony of a landscape, we adopt a distinct attitude toward the ambient world. We then allow ourselves to be taken, without haste and without any effort of analytical appreciation, by the manifold impressions reaching us. We take our time to taste the warmth of the air, the vividness of the colours, the fragrance of the trees, and the texture of the stones. It is similar to the way we taste a poem or a melody; we abandon ourselves to the succession of words and the coming and going of tones. We listen to a sonnet by Milton or a string quartet by Beethoven and take pleasure in their sense of play, partly because of their rhymes or tones, partly because of their lifting above what we call the "earnestness of life" and into the realm of *don gratuit*. Whether we are listeners or performers, we playfully receive their rhythm and harmonious sonorities as a gift and come to establish a more intimate and more personal relation to their artistic forms. By eliminating the distance separating us from the object, we linger on a temporal segment that, as it were, we lift out from our usual becoming and enjoy for its own sake.

Hamvas's book contains much more than just some indications about wines, and answers to the questions of how and when one should drink. He sees his meditations as a "prayer book for atheists" and honours wine as a symbol of God's presence. He also deals with a burning philosophical question, the sickness of abstract life. Living abstractly means, for this erudite polymath, this: to perceive and determine objects, people, actions, and values solely in relation to a single idea. Non-inclusive and brooking no contradiction, the abstract person neglects or rejects everything that lies beyond the realm defined by his conceptualizing. The uncertain, uncontrollable, and imperfect are also his worst enemies. He distrusts sensory experiences and lacks humour, serenity, and a healthy capacity for spontaneous improvisation and enjoyment. The best remedy for this sickness, Hamvas suggests, is what he calls the immediate life – a life understood as a gift, a life that asserts the intrinsic value of concrete realities and consents to these realities: a life that gives someone good conscience, quietude, understanding, and happiness. "Only one medicine can help: to live for the moment. To fall in love with the first beautiful woman, without any delay, to eat well, to walk among flowers, to go to live in the pine forest, to listen to music, to admire paintings, and to drink wine, wine, and always wine."[14]

If we accomplish our daily tasks guided only by the principles of usefulness and expedience, we usually find ourselves ahead of ourselves. Understandably, we are unwilling to live for the moment; we overlook it in our haste to reach our aim or the next event. Our thoughts and actions are fashioned above all by something that will occur in the future: a meeting we have to attend, a device we need to repair, a flight we have to catch. What the future has in store for us dominates the scene of the present. Our habitual actions, as well as the institutions that prescribe the form and timing of these actions, serve to secure predictability and expedience.

When, on the other hand, all our utilitarian aspirations recede into the background at least for a while, and the obligation to secure life's everyday needs no longer exerts its pressure on us, we are freed to consciously redirect our gaze from the future and give our attention solely to the present. The present is then opened up for activities that are ends in themselves – activities such as listening to a piano recital, chatting with an acquaintance, strolling through the streets, or contemplating a scenic view. All these experiences have something in common: they allow us to live fully in the present and enjoy whatever the present offers. When we truly and disinterestedly enjoy a captivating conversation and a glass of claret in a wine-happy company, we hold our usual means-end relations and the corresponding forward-directed attitude in abeyance. The present is no longer a stepping-stone toward specific objectives located in the future. It does not fade away or lose its fleeting character, but receives a sort of intense and satisfying extension. We sometimes have the pleasant impression that time does not move at all; nothing seems to move, even though we are surrounded by living and dynamic real-ities. If time stops advancing, the reason is not the loss of its articulation and value in relation to the future and the past, but our enlarged awareness of a duration that is complete in itself and requires no broadening backward or forward. In this singular moment of our existence, we live and are lived, we seize something and we are seized by something, we are active and receptive in the presence of the thing that holds our attention: the wine, the words and tones of our interlocutor, the landscape.

We feel the same sense of gratuitous intimacy and liberation from the passing of time when we stroll, wandering blithely into the countryside or through the streets of our neighbourhood. We advance slowly, without any purpose or obligation and, again, take pleasure in the relation of discreet familiarity with the surroundings. Strolling differs from going for a walk, which is often dictated by a pragmatic concern or a health-related objective. When we walk, we plan to cover a certain distance on a road or a path by adopting a steady pace. When we stroll, we wander aimlessly, taking irreg-ular steps, going forward as well as turning back to a place we have just left, making frequent stops here and there and responding to momentary impressions. We see things and people without making a strenuous effort of discovery; our eyes remain discreet and make no attempt to reach what is beyond appearances. "The excess of vigilance hinders the stroll," wrote Sansot.[15] We meander down the street in a state of "controlled somnolence" rather than with a "critical vision" of things, which, as we have seen, is prom-inent in a certain type of humour. In this state of reverie, we are attentive to a certain pregnant atmosphere and taste a particular style, a distinctive affective character, which comes through to us via the perception of mate-rial realities, houses, shops, streets, squares, parks, trees, but which is not identical with them. These realities have specific purposes and functions and follow each other with their particular appearance and usage in a rhythmic manner. But the "emotional essence," the "spirit" of a city, hovers above and between them, is diffused throughout the buildings and the people who live or work in them. We take in an indelible impression of this quality of life in a state of alert receptivity. The joy of the aimless stroll arises out of this global emotional experience, which wields some influence on the movement but does not stifle the feeling of being free and unconstrained, and does not force the senses to focus only on certain facets of the ambient world and remain closed to others.[16]

Strolling with ease while contemplating things with unconfined glances reveals another aspect of the attitude of *gratuité*. Let us think for a moment of the energetic walking of the person delivering our mail or taking an envelope from one side of a campus to another. One does not expect this person to introduce all sorts of imaginative variations into his movements. One expects him or her to carry out the prescribed task with the maximum of efficiency and economy, without wasting time and energy. The walking steps are measured and the corresponding amount of work defined according to the objectively defined itinerary. The person delivering our mail walks without looking around and perhaps even without thinking about anything. It is, of course, possible to cover the same distance in an entirely different manner. We could introduce rhythmic variations and nuances into our movement and through the movement express our momentary feelings, insights, and desires. Our steps, then, would take place without any purposeful planning or control, making rom for unconcerned and playful improvisation and allowing a flexible attitude toward the direction we take, the distance we cover, or the time we devote to the overall experience. This flexibility means being able to vary our tempo, stop whenever we like, make detours, and above all, to add all sorts of exploratory and seemingly useless movements. We often initiate and carry out measureless and superfluous movements of this nature as responses to the prevailing atmosphere: to the comings and goings of people around us, to a house or a tree we would like to leisurely contemplate, or to the intensity of our feelings. As we saunter with ease and explore selected parts of a town or a park or a cemetery, our movements and gestures show the mark of "playful luxury," which is, according to Buytendijk, one of the characteristics of children's play.[17]

The phenomenon of luxury is often treated today with a certain reluctance, if not with aversion or outright rejection. A person living with two of the seven deadly sins, greed and gluttony, values opulent mansions, showy cars, and fine restaurants. In professional and private contexts, one often hears that a family or a company "cannot afford such a luxury." Luxury is associated with the privilege of the few, with avoidable excess, lavishness, even waste, with frivolous accessories or behaviour, with glamorous yet futile possessions.

Luxury is a concept that we should apply with caution since it is gauged in relation to something else. Luxury does not stand alone; it is an addition to something in relation to which it exists as a desirable or undesirable reality.

A luxurious car consists of parts that are additional in relation to the basic structure that makes a car a car and as such a commonly understood means of transport. At one point in the past, perhaps, an addition was as an occasional luxury in relation to the basic structure. If, over time, this addition is included as a necessary part of the structure, it is, clearly, no longer seen as a dispensable luxury. A specific context also justifies or forbids the use of the term. For Sir Ernest Shackleton and the five other Antarctic explorers who took the perilous boat journey seeking rescue for their companions, the "glorious bath" that they enjoyed on their arrival at the island of South Georgia was a luxury. What F.A. Worsley, one of the sailors, praised as a luxury in an inhospitable context is for us today, under normal conditions, an almost unnoticed part of our daily routine.[18]

Luxury, perceived or produced by a play attitude is something useless, gratuitous yet also fulfilling, rewarding, enriching. Luxury is something added to life's necessities without being indispensable and vital. It is noticed, savoured, and nursed with delight. It brings to our everyday existence either a momentary satisfaction or a profound and lasting feeling of plenitude and joy. In the presence of a particular and simple action accomplished in the spirit of luxury, we might even declare, that without that fine additional gesture, our existence would be poorer. We might even say that it is one of the cherished things that make our life worth living. An honest and friendly praise added to a greeting, a flower brought to someone on a visit, a fine choral performance included in a graduation ceremony are heartwarming acts of luxury brought to our everyday lives. Accompanying someone home is the sort of generous deed, accomplished in the spirit of play, that can brighten the beneficiary's life in a moment of need. Robert Spaemann rightly declared that actions of that sort "make life worthwhile."[19] Although, in their forms, these actions do not appear playful at all, a play attitude of *gratuité* nevertheless animates their authors and mobilizes them into adding luxury to a lived experience.

Luxurious acts, conceived and accomplished out of an attitude of *gratuité*, are ornaments that we also value beyond the artistic sphere and see as an indispensable part of our lives. Their function is to embellish a thing or an act, to make it more pleasing to the senses, and, by doing so, enhance their being. An ornament added to something may increase our perception of its intrinsic dignity. To achieve a fitting result, the ornament must be designed and added with a fine sense of suitability, good taste, and a keen awareness of what is appropriate. An ornament of that quality does not serve to distract our vision, to alleviate uneasy feelings, or to hide undesired aspects of a thing. Before an ornament can be designed and added, the object in question has already been recognized as worthy of admiration and love. Indeed, as Jacques Dewitte has pointed out, a "loving intention" expressed towards something that we take into our caring hands presides over every genuine act of orna-mentation.[20] One might see in the ornament only a useless and superfluous supplement appended to a reality already possessing merit and value in itself. Yet, it is also possible to see an ornament as an "imperative necessity" and to sense the pathic influence of a missing, still non-existent decorative addition. Because we view a building or a piece of clothing with love and care, and measure its form and value against a standard other than what is perceived as a strictly functional and useful reality, we gladly respond to its invitation to add decorative motifs.

Still, adding an ornament to a door, for example, does not mean that we can overlook the functionality of that important movable barrier. Our sense of aptness needs to take into account its everyday use. We must see how the added ornament affects the movement from one space to another. If the adorned door adequately fulfils its purpose, then both the onlooker standing at a distance and the person passing through the door will find it appealing.

Just as an apartment, an office, a library, a shop, a building, or a car calls for, and admits, ornament, likewise, the manifold activities and relations of our everyday lives aspire to be enriched with embellishment. Our daily in-teractions with people also require some sort of enrichment, however slight this might be. Whenever we meet another person, at work, in a stores or at an airport, we sense that our verbal exchange cannot be limited to the strict minimum. Before expressing a wish or making a request, we begin by voic-ing a greeting and by asking simple questions such as "how are you?" We address the other person by using a formal salutation or even by making a detour in the conversation, taking the time to ask a question, perhaps to offer well-deserved praise or the wish of success for whatever the other person is trying to accomplish. Of course, there is always the risk of turning the com-munication into an artificial and phoney exchange of empty words. And it is always possible to put aside the formalities and, in the manner of a customs or police officer, proceed in a direct and expedient manner. In his reflections on courtesy, Guardini has warned about the pernicious consequences of the diminution of courteous behaviour in our lives.[21] His warning is relevant to our time, when people tend to eschew courteous detours in the numerous instantaneous text messages they write every day. When formalities are treated as superfluous and a waste of time, human life as a whole is "impoverished and coarsened." Although written many years ago, Guardini's caveat about "life deprived of the 'extras'" rings more true than ever today. It deplores the evanescence of what I have called the luxurious deeds and little ornaments of everyday life, and links the "moral degeneration" of an entire population to the "lowering of the tone of everyday communication."[22]

In the absence of an attitude that perceives and values what is beyond the realm of the utilitarian and impersonal, and which fosters and cultivates gratuitous interactions, social virtues such as politeness, courtesy, civility, or kindness and tolerance will hardly be able to find their expression in our lives. As Helmuth Plessner has convincingly emphasized, ethics is not simply a matter of obedience to some externally imposed and rationally approved set of directives, principles, rules, conventions, and values. Human beings cannot, and should not, act only according to the dictates of their social conscience; they have the need and right to rely on other resources than their reason, which tells them what is good and proper. There are decisions that require one to venture beyond the limits of rationally approved norms and regulations. There are actions that are prompted by luminous and creative intuition, by a keen sense of the exceptional. Plessner rejects the idea of defining the ethical sphere solely by the respect accorded a prevalent code of ethics. On rational grounds alone, gratuitous kindness would find no justification; it is generated by a feeling of sympathy or love rather than by obedience to certain values and norms. Similarly, when people are required to do "great things," their behaviour is often inspired by the "spirit of luxury."[23]

The same spirit presides over actions of lesser magnitude. The delicacy of tact is a form of sensibility that, in the absence of a well-designed ethical code, plays a pivotal role in interpersonal relations. Tact is a fine sense for nuance, timing, and proportion that tells us what to do and how to behave when rules, principles, and norms fail to provide us with a reliable and trustworthy guidance. To be sure, the wisdom of tact helps us respond adequately to unforeseen situations and choose the correct, decent, and appropriate form of behaviour. It tells us, for instance, what and how to refuse something politely when we are approached by an unexpected and unacceptable demand. Tact is also an active quality that suggests surprising initiatives: creating a friendly atmosphere with the help of humour, giving a well-chosen gift that brings unanticipated joy to someone's life, intuiting someone's need to talk and listening with genuine interest, without offending or intruding. Tact is, then, the virtue which, out of generosity and kindness, creates peaceful and respectful communications among members of a smaller or larger community; it nurtures the "culture of apparent superfluity," and cultivates the "solace and elevation of life."[24]

In one of his "spiritual letters," the recently rediscovered Italian philosopher Giuseppe Rensi refers, in connection to the child's play, to a state of serious and gratuitous engagement. The attitude of the child toward his play is seen by Rensi as a model for adults to follow.

> The child who plays views his play as a serious thing and is devoted to his play with the most earnest eagerness (to the point of getting carried away and coming to blows) but always bearing in mind the precept that it is not a substantial reality and the world of play is not the world of real life. There is the solution. We need to have, in our life, something similar to what play means for children: something, as a serious thing that interests us, something, to which we devote ourselves with the most earnest eagerness and, something that at the same time guarantees us that *it has no essential importance*."[25]

Rensi mentions the manner with which we used to engage with the world in our childhood. We turned to all aspects of our play, the toys, rules, the forms of movement, with utmost care and concentration, with "earnest eagerness." I have already mentioned the ardent desire of children to accept attentively and follow correctly the prescribed rules and codes of any game, however absurd and provisory they may have seemed. How much joy we felt when, at our tender age, we were imitating and idealizing the world as we saw it and as we wanted to see it. No matter the degree of our enchantment, the return to the real world was, eventually, an inevitable necessity.

Rensi recommends the conscious reprise of the attitude of child's. We should devote ourselves wholeheartedly, he suggests, to a chosen activity; we should mobilize all our energies to practise an art form, to pursue a hobby, or to organize social gatherings. Yet, however seriously and passionately we play the violin or practise swimming or spend countless hours embellishing a home garden or a public park, these activities should never have, for us, an "essential importance."

What does it mean to having or not have an "essential importance"? To be essential is to be an indispensable constituent of a reality: wheels for a bicycle, wings for an airplane, oxygen for human beings. What is essential, in a strict sense, for humans is what we need for living. Essential to life are air, water, food, clothing, a place where we eat, rest, sleep and where we are protected from inclement weather. In a broader sense, fulfilling human relations, a sense of well-being, and something that brings to an activity a meaning and not merely a purpose are among the indispensable elements of our lives.

There is, of course, no definitive agreement among people regarding what constitutes essential or non-essential realities in a wider sense. For some, listening to classical or jazz music is an essential part of their daily lives; for others it is not. For some, doing physical exercise every morning is not essential; for others it is.

The "non-essentials" of life are things in the absence of which we may find our existence uneventful and barely tolerable, though their absence does not impede us from continuing to live: pursuing a particular leisure activity, visiting public gardens, or being a member of a club, an association, or a political party. Non-essentials are those elements that, with time, have become customary and widely accepted parts of our lives, but from which we are able to part if some reason – a modification of our financial, health, or social conditions – demands such a release.

Having no essential value also means, in this context, that a thing or a pursuit has no useful purpose. We tinker with radio or computer parts, paint portraits, or take photographs with great delight. We undertake these activities regardless of whether we receive from them any practical benefit, financial reward or social recognition. We assemble computers and apply paint to canvas for the sake of the activity itself and not for the gains that we expect to obtain. The non-essential activity that we accomplish with utmost passion is self-sufficient and free of utilitarian concerns.

Why does Rensi view a play attitude as a "solution"? And if a solution, for what kind of problem?

The first aspect of the problem evoked here is the absence of motivation and desire to fully give oneself, with consistency and enthusiasm, to an endeavour: a worthy civic cause, a domain of study, a specific vocation. We may think here of students who enrol in university studies with the sole purpose of training for a job. Most of today's universities respond to their need to find satisfactory employment but fail to show them how to pursue a perhaps less lucrative but more fulfilling path in the arts or sciences, or prepare them to choose a life of passionate dedication to an uncommon aim. Such students seem to lack a sense of higher purpose that would guide them to a resolute course of action committed to the opportunities and duties conveyed by their ideals.

A second and no less crucial aspect is the inability to free oneself from the perspective of usefulness in order to be able to do something for the sheer pleasure of moving, creating, and being in touch with a material form, and not solely for reaching a useful end. In William James's essay on relaxation, from which I have already quoted, James spoke of the inhibitive influence of the "egoistic preoccupation about results." He makes the comparison between two workers: the first is excessively careful and preoccupied only about the result and, accordingly, accomplishes his work in a state of tension and of anxiety, and the second is a "relaxed and easy worker, who is in no hurry, and quite thoughtless most of the while of consequences." In truth, adds James, the relaxed worker is the "efficient worker."[26] The question James raised is similar to the problem that Rensi addressed: how to teach someone to focus with dedicated attention on the accomplishment of a task and at the same time remain unconcerned about its practical outcome. Combining concentration with relaxation is, in the eyes of other thinkers and educators, the key to reaching proficiency and satisfaction in any field. It is through concentration that we can immerse ourselves in an activity and fend off all external disturbances. And it is through relaxation that we remove the barriers of our calculating consciousness and allow the unrestricted functioning of our bodily powers. We gradually realize that effort and the serious practice of an art are necessary, but not anxious effort and not nervous and tense practice.[27]

It seems to me that Rensi's solution finds distinct and inspiring expression in the play attitude of the amateur, who, as we have seen before, is not bound to professional standards of performance. Amateurs sing, paint, write poems, and carve wood or stone into forms at their own leisure and with a total unconcern about the financial and social import of their achievements. Guided by an impractical vision, they neither seek public adulation nor receive critical recognition; and they reap no material benefits from their inherent and learned technical skills.

We see lovers of music coming together in someone's house or in a cultural centre, after their working hours, to play tunes from diverse times and cultures, and to invent new melodies of their own. While professional musicians perform with precision and polish, amateurs play their pieces with enthusiasm and gaiety. Amateurs are pleased to rediscover the playful character of music. Whether they make music alone or in a small ensemble, they play in the exact sense of the word. Free from the imperative of flawless and expedient performance, they yield spontaneously to the inspiration of the moment and bring subtle ornamentations and slight deviations to their play. Amateurs approach any art form with purposeless ingenuity and favourably complement any deficiencies of specialized expertise with a sense of luxury and genuine receptivity to a wide range of forms. They benefit from a familiarity with various styles and a sensitivity to the elements uniting diverse musical communities.[28]

There is one more reason to praise the amateur. In his foreword to Sophie Deroisin's inspiring book *Le Prince de Ligne*, Simon Leys accords a certain prominence to being "an amateur in the deepest, most complete and most fruitful sense of the word."[29] Although without a specialized profession and qualification, the prince, an amateur courtier, had numerous praiseworthy qualities: he pursued a wide variety of activities for their own sake; he acted with detachment, enthusiasm, and nonchalance, under the inspiration of the moment; he was open-minded, acting everywhere as a foreign visitor and marvelling at things at every touch and turn; he was courageous, taking risks in both physical and emotional ways. Leys adds that, for someone practising a range of disciplines with an "exquisite inexpertness," "at bottom there is only one art that matters, and that is the art of life."[30]

8

Play Aptitudes and the Art of Living

Following up on the concluding remark of the previous chapter, we may safely assert that, for individuals who address life's greater tasks and everyday events with an attitude of play, the art of living matters. They know that responding with humour to an incident at home is no less important than rationally resolving a problem at work. They feel that their lives would be stale and boring without the salutary tension produced by the risk of declaring love or the lightness and ease experienced while holding something of their creative powers in reserve. They have come to realize that the transient adoption of play attitude is one of the fundamental presuppositions of right and creative living; in addition, it offers one of the best ways to enjoy life.

The gratifying art of living develops through the gradual acquisition and consistent use of qualities and virtues that give a sense of plenitude, a feeling of harmony with the world. Practitioners of the art of living may take initiatives or participate in activities and say as they do so: "I have the impression of living a more fulfilled life." Practising an art such as painting or gardening, enjoying a leisure activity, acquiring greater knowledge of a chosen subject, and performing volunteer work in a community are some of the ways of living a more complete life. The art of living also finds expression in the level of competence reached in one or more of these domains. It may involve knowing, for instance, how to conduct a delicate conversation, when to speak, when to listen, when to yield, when to hold onto a conviction, when to broach sensitive issues with warm humour, or when to communicate tersely dry facts. It may consist of deciding when to leave an unpropitious living condition, how to ride on the flow of time or seize the right and opportune moment to introduce a change in one's existence, how to face the uncertainties of tomorrow with quiet courage. It may imply intuiting when to refrain from action and remain, for a while, a calm and patient spectator of unfolding events. The art of living entails the practice of certain dispositions and the uninhibited manifestation of certain aptitudes that either prevail in specific domains or pervade one's whole existence and fashion an enduring lifestyle. A physician who is kind and generous in interactions with patients, for instance, may nonetheless have difficulty transferring this excellence and expressing it in other areas of everyday life. Each domain has its unspoken rules and undergoes constant change. What seems to be appropriate at one time may prove inadequate at another.

The art of living does not derive from hard-won professional expertise. Extensive knowledge does not guarantee the practice of courtesy or benevolence in everyday life. We have all met people who know everything in their professions yet fail to relate to their fellow human beings with any degree of social grace. They soar high at work among their colleagues and yet sink low when ordering their meal in a restaurant. Yet, as Alain maintained, "there is an art of life in which politeness, properly understood, is almost everything and indeed is everything."[1] It was a similar conviction that prompted Vaclav Havel to say that a graduate degree in political science does not necessarily grant the ability to comprehend problems as well as human characters and to tailor one's own words and acts to the requirements of a given situation.[2] Educational institutions seldom facilitate the acquisition of the ability to make a decision autonomously in the face of powerful social influences. If learning this and other abilities takes place in schools, the gain is most likely an unwitting side effect that is happily produced when a teacher is able to evoke in students a shared passion for a subject or when students have the opportunity to converse unreservedly with each other between classes. Students rarely acquire from textbooks a sense of how to welcome a foreign student, how to show tolerance or compassion once peace has been declared between conflicting parties, or how to respond to the distress and isolation of a fellow human being. In short, the qualities and principles of the art of living are internalized primarily thanks to concrete activities carried on outside the formal and traditional educational context.

I maintain that the attitude of play is central to the art of living and as such, it gets its vitality from particular human qualities. Its fundamental manifestations – pathic receptivity, ease, risk, humour, *gratuité* – are grounded in human qualities to such an extent that they form an inseparable unity. Hartmann stressed this underlying relation in his statement that: "sense of humour is a genuine aesthetic stance, but one always resting on an *ethos*. This *ethos* must, of course, be summoned up, must, as it were, be erected from within."[3] *Ethos* is understood here as an abiding moral quality consisting of being able to look at oneself without inhibition. Those who possess this quality are best able to express humour or to display a receptivity to humour. In the sentence quoted earlier, we have seen that Benveniste pointed to the same relation: "playing means forgetting the useful, beneficially submitting oneself to the forces that real-life conditions curb and harm." He saw in play the possibility of leaving behind all utilitarian aims and of reviving *forces* that have been silenced and marginalized.[4] When we adopt a play attitude, we draw on these forces and allow them a satisfying mode of expression. As long as they sustain the attitude of play, we might call them "play-aptitudes," knowing well at the same time that they may wield their influence in experiences in which the play attitude no longer has any relevance or justification.

What are these qualities or forces – these play-aptitudes? In the preceding chapters, I have hinted at the human qualities of availability, spontaneity, and purposeless freedom. I have also mentioned the ability to face uncertainty and the art of seeing things from a superior point of view. I now contend that these qualities contribute to the adoption and development of a form of play attitude. Their influence is wide-ranging and, in my opinion, central to the art of living.

We recall that children readily adopt a responsive attitude in the presence of objects in their environment that exhibit, for them, an expressive and inviting presence. They convert all sorts of activities and objects into situations of play. Adults also have the ability to restore a living and animated world and recover the tendency to playfulness in their behaviour. But in order to create a new and distinctive relation to people and things, they need to envisage their momentary obligations and duties both with an earnest sense of responsibility and with an unconcerned and liberal frame of mind.

Earlier in this book I have referred to the way the common experience of seeing a ball rolling toward us in a public park and responding to it highlights the nature of this responsiveness. We all know from our own experience how irresistible the desire is to catch and throw or to kick the ball back to someone. Of course, it is always possible to ignore the ball's appeal. If we happen to walk with a preoccupied mindset or if we want to hold fast to our dignified posture, we just mind our own business and let the ball go by; we choose to be "impregnable" and remain tied to our aloof and indifferent attitude. If we become *available* and opt to modify our behaviour, we happily return the ball and enjoy the pleasant sensation of kicking or throwing it. We respond to similar kinds of persuasive "invitations" in situations in which we modify our planned activity and spontaneously adapt to a suddenly appearing demand.

Availability is the human quality that enables us to be open and receptive to appeals addressed to us by fellow human beings and by the things we encounter in our daily existence. We are available when we no longer perceive a lamp, a piece of paper, or a table as neutral and indifferent objects that silently serve our practical quotidian needs, but as things that tell us something, communicating an invitation to our rational mind and sensitive body. If we are available, we can allow ourselves to hear the language of things, to be affected by their immediate and intense radiance, and to respond to their palpable suggestions in full freedom and ease.

While playing, we actively turn to the animated presence of a swing or a ball and spontaneously respond to its invitation. By adopting a play attitude outside the sphere of play, we find ourselves able to perceive, and yield to, the call of things. We become sensitive to their suggestions and expressive qualities.

I have also pointed out that, among our many encounters with people and things, we gladly, or perhaps somewhat apprehensively, single out interactions that convey new possibilities. Availability in such instances consists of welcoming possibilities, facilitating their realization, and living with the risk of failing. By acting upon these possibilities, selecting or discarding them, we introduce changes into our lives. For these changes to take place, we need to take a distance from ourselves and from our habitual ways of perceiving and doing things, in order to make the selected possibilities our own and, through their realization, to let them exert their effective influence on our being. We may, then, consciously revise our future plans, modify our lifestyle, or espouse a new vocation.

In reflecting on the concept of availability (*disponibilité*), Gabriel Marcel refers to the phenomenon of hospitality, which implies responding to a request, sharing a personal world with guests, offering them a place of rest, inviting them to participate in one's own activities, opening a home and a part of oneself, in the spirit of *gratuité*, to a foreign presence. Giving something of oneself to a guest, caring about his or her comfort and well-being, transforming one's home and making changes in one's habitual pattern of living are all at the heart of fraternal hospitality, made possible by the quality of availability.[5]

I would suggest that many creative solutions grow out of, and benefit from, the quality of availability. When someone decides to create a tool of some kind of material – wood, stone, or metal – the shape of the tool emerges obviously from the interaction between the maker's mental conception and the characteristics of the material. It would be a mistake, however, to think that the work is guided only by the mental image of the tool, which highlights its form and practical purposes. When the process of making a tool leaves room for creative modification, a fruitful dialogue takes place between the obedient hand, carrying out the directives of a mental conception, and the available hand, responding to the "suggestions" of the material. Psychologist of art Rudolf Arnheim, in an article on the perception and handling of art objects, quotes the observations of two Italian anthropologists on the shepherds of Sardinia. They noticed that the shepherds introduced into the act of carving tools an "element of playfulness" with an attitude of what they describe as "affectionate carelessness." Accepting the obstacles and surprises inherent in the material, they are prepared to depart from their initial conceptions, creating one-of-a-kind objects to this day.[6]

A playful and easy-going availability may of course nurture creativity in the everyday lives of ordinary people in less remote contexts as well. A particular task or challenge often requires a disposition to remain receptive to a new idea or a new way of doing things, deviating from a preconceived plan, and weighing the value of each proposed novelty. This sort of creativity does not necessarily lead to brilliant discoveries or inventions; nor does it produce remarkable and much admired works of art or athletic feats. It shows itself at unexpected moments such as when a problem finds its long-awaited solution in an immediate and instantaneous manner. Students blocked in their effort of formulating the conclusion of a term paper or the central questions of a dissertation may come suddenly and surprisingly, in flashes of breakthrough, to the so-called rush of ideas when conscious tension gives way to unconstrained relaxation, the active will to quiet receptivity. Similarly, professionals working in urban planning, mechanical engineering, or marketing may have their own "Eureka moments." They may receive startling insights while casually conversing with friends or colleagues or leisurely doodling on sketches. When additional new ideas, solutions, flashes of insight, unusual forms, or unsuspected combinations of cause and effect spontaneously emerge on the heels of an initial discovery, they experience instants of expansive plenitude.

It is worth emphasizing the central role that an attitude of relaxed availability plays in every creative endeavour. The suggestion to alternate active and receptive states is just as relevant today as it was years ago, when art therapist Florence Cane placed it at the heart of her theory of creativity. She suggested that, if an art student is stymied by an insurmountable difficulty, he should throw himself on a couch, close his eyes, and let the image in his mind speak to him. In this quiet, dreamy, receptive state, the pathic relation to the image will eventually bring clarification, renewed energy, and unforeseen solutions. "The darkness, the quiet, the withdrawal, all help the boy to find the next step."[7] A similar kind of creative proficiency is available to us all, she continued, when, fully aware how futile it is to force an issue, we combine effort with repose – acting by lingering, doing by not-doing. "The idea of consciously – rhythmically – alternating the process of giving out and taking in is so simple that it seems obvious, but few people make use of it."[8]

To our activities undertaken in the spirit of play, *spontaneity* brings exuberance, lavishness, and a superabundance of energy. Whether working on joinery or taking part in a communal dance, we have the impression of drawing on the dynamism of life within us, being carried by an élan. Our movements unfold with suppleness, luxury, and grace, abandoning functional sobriety and calculated economy. Spontaneous actions make an awareness and display of a joyously and profusely functioning body possible. A body inspired by spontaneity moves with admirable proficiency on autopilot, so to speak, and this, perhaps above all else, is its most important contribution to the art of living. No longer is the body perceived as if something separate; it is neither an instrument to manipulate nor an obstacle to overcome. Calling on its experience in an effortless display of powers and possibilities, the body exhibits poise, invention, and intelligence, because it follows its own impulses and desires, sets its own rhythm, responds with skill to any perturbation, and explores new and unusual solutions. In a word, it does what it feels is the right thing to do. Philosophers, psychologists, psychiatrists, biologists, writers, and artists have drawn our attention to the surprising knowledge of the body which, thanks to its previously learned skills and natural spontaneity, is able to move with ease, producing a great variety of forms of its own accord.[9] We all have experienced, under diverse circumstances, agreeable moments when our willed determination to move in a certain way yields to our body's own intentions and imponderable energies and our responses and explorations occur effortlessly with alertness and ease.

Spontaneity also plays a role in interpersonal exchanges. When an action is spontaneously addressed to a fellow human being, it is carried out without calculation, hesitation, or expectation of reciprocity. Spontaneity instigates the praise that a coach extends, in the heat of a game, to an athlete in need of valuation and of approval. Spontaneity extends the helping hand that a passerby lends, without hesitation or deliberation, to a person who accidently falls off his bicycle. These and other such benevolent actions are accomplished with no regard to the possible self-satisfaction of their authors; they exclude ulterior and selfish motives. The praise or helping hand that we offer another person asserts its intrinsic life-enhancing value independently of any approval or expression of gratitude.

Perhaps I have placed too much emphasis on the rightness and appropriateness of spontaneity. This quality applies well to an athletic or artistic performance or to an illustration that a speaker advances in order to make a speech livelier and more concrete. Can we notice spontaneity in other spheres of our lives? We might take a risk about a career or a place of living spontaneously and in a spirit of play, without assessing, weighing, imagining the possible consequences of our decision over days and weeks. We may simply seize one life-defining possibility and discard another equally alluring one without constraint or fruitless pondering. In retrospect, we might come to regret our chosen vocation or new home and start to treat spontaneity with suspicion. We might for a short while chose to favour prudence and act with caution after lengthy calculation. However, if we put aside our disappointment and maintain our attitude of play, we may find ourselves attracted to spontaneity as a guiding "image, perspective, and aspiration" of our life.[10]

The phenomenon of decision-making brings to the fore an acknowledgment that we live with a vivid *sense of uncertainty*. In a moment of selecting one of the two excluding possibilities, we are in a quandary, unable to assess the outcome of our decision with clarity or certainty. Being exposed to the risk of failing, and anticipating the future with doubt are both elements of the decision-making process. We must face the possible consequences of our decisions – the possibility of living with failure and enduring the discomfort and sometimes even lasting pain that failure may bring us.

To be sure, some would prefer to eliminate from their lives any experiences that involve states of uncertainty. Social institutions – with their rules, laws, habits, and behaviour patterns – can ensure a much-desired predictability of human behaviour and communal events. They alleviate the obligation of making decisions and dispel the corresponding disquiet of what Straus calls "living in the provisional." They tend to minimize the openness of the future by telling us in advance the outcome of various experiences and, when the results are nevertheless unexpected, by fitting them into measures, policies, and procedures already in place. Yet undertaking an activity with an acute sense of uncertainty can be a welcome part of a professional life as well as a particular leisure pursuit. As we have earlier seen, numerous adepts of so-called risk sports and travellers to hidden parts of the world delight in surrendering themselves to the unpredictable and to the correlating risk. Like gamblers who relish living for a short time in a state of uncertainty, people undertaking activities in a playful manner – a new research endeavour, travel to an unfamiliar land, work accomplished beyond one's training and experience – can also feel the thrill of not being able to know in advance the outcome of their decisions.

We may compare these and other similar experiences to listening to a pianist's live recital. Will the performance convey assurance or hesitancy, brilliance or blandness? Will the playing flow smoothly or will it be spoiled by false notes or slips of memory? The philosopher Vladimir Jankélévitch compares the virtuoso's playing to an "acrobatic play,"[11] which, with its heightened degree of dramatic tension, is "a reduced image of human life." The pianist's hands bounce, rebound, and fall with elegance on the right note. Moreover, listeners may welcome the uncertainty of a gap between what a musical score prescribes and what an artist proposes during a concert hall interpretation. The perpetual variability of individual interpretation always depends on the musician's vitality and energy in the moment, without which a performance is nothing but a mechanical and artificial production. The playful tendency of the musician to respond with relative freedom to the invitations of tones and numerous momentary variables (audience, acoustics, or instrument) is another magnet that draws certain listeners to live concerts. The unpredictability of live performances makes them attractive and offers a more fulfilling artistic experience than the flawless yet bland and non-ludic interpretations available on recordings.

These examples refer to transient experiences that create the tension of unpredictability only for a limited phase of our becoming. The momentary aspect of unpredictability makes gambling or any other similar playful activity a short-lived experience. It is always possible to leave a game or a concert, to interrupt a travel or a scientific study, if the intensity of the tension becomes unbearable. We accept living with the tension of unpredictability within the continuity of our lives inasmuch as, armed with our tolerance of uncertainty, we can continue to remain open to an unknown future and let the future bring its new possibilities. In other words, however important it is to commit ourselves to the realization of habitual projects, our sense of continuity can remain receptive to possible discontinuous innovations and to the resulting possibilities of failures and disappointments. We then no longer count only on the familiarity of our surroundings and the predictability of institutional conventions; we also accept that the future, from time to time, contradicts our expectations. It means concretely that we dare to take more weighty risks and thereby envisage the possibility of a reversal of our personal and professional conditions even if no actual event suggests a turn of fortune; our health, wealth, social recognition – even freedom – can be threatened or lost from one day to the next. We admit that there is a gap between what we experience and imagine in the present and the still unknown reality that the future has in store for us; we no longer rely exclusively on protective bridges built between the present and the future with the help of careful activity management and excessive safety procedures.[12]

The corollary of a realistic and open approach to an unpredictable future is the ability to rise above our everyday life and view our actions, obligations, and human relations with equanimity. We have seen that through humour we are able to stand above our circumstances and, in a relaxed and friendly manner, put up with our fellow human beings, with all their virtues and shortcomings – and even with the dumbfounding incongruity of their actions. In a well-crafted article, Jan Linschoten stressed the paradoxical blending of dispassion and involvement in humour: "On the one hand, humour calls for a distance and a perspective; on the other hand, it creates an intimate relation to the human, an awareness of one's own humanity and other humans as they are: although absurd, it is also good and beautiful."[13] Humour, in its puzzling and enigmatic relation to human realities, presupposes a *sense of superiority* that has nothing to do with the sense of entitlement, patronizing disdain, or the aloof gaze that is prone to belittle worthy achievements and to combat and discard dissenting point of views.

"Superiority," *Überlegenheit*, is an *ethos* about which Hartmann has written with subtlety in his *Aesthetics*.[14] It consists of placing human weaknesses and flaws in a wider context together with human qualities. They then appear in such a way that contrasting inadequacies are tactfully smoothed out as if being viewed from afar. Superiority presupposes an inner peacefulness that is sensed as a person's atmosphere by all those who are exposed to it. It offers an invisible protection from the petty miseries of everyday life by becoming a force to help deal with its more severe misfortunes. Superiority of this kind is revealed, above all, in the "sense and receptivity to humour" in its varying manifestations, in the "open-mindedness" and the "inner ease" that release both humorist and auditor from compulsive inhibitions. People with a sense of humour enjoy an advantage over those who are humourless, fixed in their pedantry, rigidity, obstinacy. The greatest drawback of the humourless person is an inability to laughingly accept being the butt of a practical joke or a simple humorous remark. The most such a person can do is to put on a brave face in response to a perceived wicked game.[15]

As for its scope, the sense of superiority in Hartmann's meaning extends beyond the realm of humour. It nurtures a healthy scepticism about the roles, achievements, and aspirations that we tend to deem important and long-lasting. Fame and reputation always wax and wain. Humour fosters a detachment from usual practices and elaborated plans, and proposes spontaneous improvisations and daring risks. This detachment may take the form of a poised indifference with regard to whatever happens to us; we couldn't care less whether our undertakings yield success or failure, acquisitions or losses, recognition or rejection, or even solidarity or adversity. In this state of insouciance, our achievements or triumphs and the corresponding repose of satisfaction and self-congratulation become secondary. What matters is the activity itself, the free and disinterested giving of the self, with little concern for the result.

The French philosopher Louis Lavelle warned that "allowing ourselves to be enslaved by success" is what poses the greatest danger to our liberty: "For every success that we may achieve, in any field, is merely the triumph for the individual that we are – something from which we personally profit. But in the spiritual order, our goal is not profit but an act to be accomplished, the exercise of our capacities, not their increase, and the sacrifice of the self, which is also the fulfilment of the self."[16] For Lavelle an absence of concern, or indifference, is not an insensitive hardness of the heart; it is a charitable feeling that raises a person to a higher level and achieves a "victory over self-love." It abolishes prejudices and preferences, thereby nurturing the aptitude of putting great and small things on the same plane and the capacity to see value and meaning in even the smallest among them. Those who recognize the importance of seemingly negligible events will not place emphasis only on notable achievements and on the ensuing reputation and applause. They know that, if accomplished with resoluteness and monk-like devotion, the most commonplace activity also brings profound contentment, and that, regardless of their magnitude, "the finest achievements are never seen by the crowd."[17]

By focusing selflessly and unreservedly on the act itself and not being preoccupied by the result of a performance that might bring profit and recognition, our apparent indifference has an affinity with an aesthetic relation to the world. *Aesthetic responsiveness* to things is another condition of a genuine attitude of play and, in my opinion, is central to the art of living. As Martine Mauriras-Bousquet has expressed it, we come to adopt a playful attitude when we learn "to desire aesthetically the world, the world around us."[18]

The phenomenon of an aesthetic preoccupation and interest is a huge topic. Let us content ourselves here with a few remarks about this capacity, which underlies the attitude of play so beneficially to be adopted in our everyday lives.

It is clear that, whenever we marvel at the beauty of a landscape or a well-designed garden, walk around or even touch a sculpture, or listen attentively to a Chopin mazurka, we create an aesthetic relation to an object. These objects present distinctive qualities – unity, harmony, order, balance, complexity, proportion, clarity, rhythm, fittingness, surprise, or rightness – and we use these terms and others as we justify the intensification of our awareness. When we perceive, in the countryside, the midsummer flowering plants, the circling birds, and the humming bees, the source of our aesthetic enjoyment is the harmony of living beings. We do not invoke this kind of value judgment only in a museum or a concert hall, or when we are moved by the beauty of a landscape. We apprehend aesthetic values when we let our fingers follow the curved contours of an old car (Jaguar E-Type, for example), approach a decorative wooden staircase, take a fine calligraphy pen in hand, or even relish a graceful goal-scoring movement accomplished by a player of our favourite team.

How does one establish an aesthetic relation to things and people within an everyday milieu and perceive the above-mentioned values? What sort of attitude is conducive to an aesthetic experience? One way of evoking an aesthetic experience is to interrupt or halt an activity and to suspend for a time the will required to attend to a previously identified aim. Someone walking hurriedly along a street to arrive in time for a previously arranged appointment most likely fails to appreciate the intricate and delicate details on a building. A person entering a church with the firm intention of spending the next fifteen minutes kneeling and praying fervently with bowed head will not contemplate the frescoes and arches in a state of wonder. The perception of both persons glides over even the most beautiful of objects and notices only what seem to be relevant to the intention to reach a destination or express one's devotion. The aesthetic relation, on the other hand, is aided by the attitude that allows one to stop and dwell on something. Here is an example given by George H. Mead in his essay on aesthetic experience: "The artisan who stops to sense the nice perfection of a tool or a machine has interrupted its use to appreciate it, and is in an aesthetic mood. He is not interested in its employment, he is enjoying it."[19] Thanks to the interruption of the activity and detachment from all utilitarian aims, the perception of the artisan becomes autonomous. Nevertheless, the practical usefulness of the object, which justifies its being, does not disappear completely; the artisan merely considers it, at that moment, unworthy of his attention. An aesthetic relation to an object is achieved thanks to the attitude of freeing the object from one's goal-oriented stream of interests and actions. The object is approached with an altogether new frame of mind; it is contemplated. In this context, contemplation means paying attention to an object in a state of alert receptiveness, without any effort to insert the object into a structure of means and ends.

What can occur during a moment of perception when, like an artisan, we pause and allow our senses the opportunity to receive impressions with no desire to use them in the present or to exploit them for some future purpose?

Let us suppose that we interrupt our energetic walk as we arrive at a square and decide to dwell on the sight of this large open area. We see a place of worship, a fountain, a newsstand, cafés, shops, people walking to-and-fro or sitting on benches, trees, house façades, balconies, and other architectural subtleties. We may also notice the impatient vehicles, chirping pigeons, laughing children, gossiping adults, blaring sound-systems, and other congenial or unpleasant noises. We apprehend all these things in their completeness together with the manifold connections they entertain with each other and with their proper environment. We no longer perceive isolated and selected realities that respond to our matter-of-fact interest, such as the time schedule listed at the bus stop or the newspaper with its market reports. We construct an image of the entire square and find pleasure in the picture-like sensuous form – the harmony of shapes, contours, figures, and sounds as they complement and contrast each other, the rhythm of patterns and designs, the interplay of lights and shadows, strident noises and soft sounds.[20]

I have briefly emphasized the pictorial quality of the square, the autonomous unity of the key elements of a composition, because the same liberation from practical interest may lead us to linger playfully upon other forms. We are able to brood over the sensuous appearance of things and call upon our imagination to create or break connections freely and light-heartedly, to take things apart and reunite them according to our own inclinations, not by their relation to functional matters. The same touch of playfulness may find a role in the physical activity of placing furniture, carpets, lamps, vases, or books in a room or arranging flowers and bushes in a garden according to their shapes and colours. A playful sense of form may prompt free-spirited students to create and wear clothing that mixes a variety of conspicuous colours, or to place a peculiar-looking giraffe in the midst of a presidential welcoming ceremony.

The aesthetic awareness cannot be satisfied only by contemplating forms and ordering formal relations in the imagination. We enjoy seeing and altering shapes, colours, figures, and lines because they are tied to things that make a room or a garden warm and pleasant. Likewise, we delight in meeting people whose jovial and friendly manners are true reflections of their feelings and characters.

In our everyday lives, we already perceive things with their affective characteristics. When we enter a public park or a cemetery, we notice an atmospheric quality radiating from these spaces. For the sake of gaining impartial and objective knowledge, we may eliminate the expressive quality from our conscious perception. In our aesthetic experience, however, we bring out more fully the affective quality from the perceived reality, lend animation to the inanimate, and humanize the non-human; we then gaze, for instance, at the sadness of the tree, the loneliness of the meadow, or the "dark menace of a narrow grave" (Joseph Conrad).

The aesthetic awareness, in which beyond the formal elements the emotional aspects of things also come forth, nurtures and accentuates playfulness. As I pointed out previously, people have a tendency to attribute to their cherished objects tonalities of feelings and treat these objects playfully as if they had their own "personality," their own expressive presence. With regard to this attribution of tonalities of joy or sorrow to inanimate things, Hartmann speaks of a "creative consciousness" that is "closely related to aesthetical consciousness."[21] This creative consciousness is at work when food placed on the table receives a new significance and the process of eating is enriched with visual fantasies or when the wines we taste are associated with human qualities such as reserve or smiling serenity. It also fosters humour, which highlights contrasts, brings life to a lifeless reality, cancels out our usual valuation of things, and sees in the world new wonders and life's incongruous mysteries.

I have so far considered the aesthetic experience as a relation to things and people involving disinterest in their utilitarian purposes. The experience stands out from the succession of everyday events and occurrences. We find ourselves in an "aesthetic mood" when we introduce a pause into the progress of our purposive activities, seek and reach an intense and extended awareness of the formal and emotional aspects of a reality, and dwell upon it for its own sake.

If we observe certain activities of our everyday lives, however, we realize that we may also come to enjoy an aesthetic experience even when we are absorbed in the stream of useful activities. We do not always need to take a distance from our practical interests in order to apprehend the formal and emotional facets of things and, if the situation is suitable, to perceive them playfully. In fact, if we are not troubled by distracting side issues, a wide range of objects best reveal their aesthetic qualities when we are using them. Then, we adopt, in the words of Moritz Geiger, the attitude of "contemplative using" or "contemplation during use."[22] Clothes and jewels manifest their eye-catching brilliance when they have a contact with our living bodies. Porcelains, glasses, bowls, plates, utensils can surely be seen in museums. But we may better capture their aesthetic qualities if we take them into our hands as we accomplish our worthwhile activities of eating and drinking. We may admire the beauty of a hall while we are giving a lecture there to an attentive audience; we may appreciate the architectural splendour of a building while we undertake its renovation; we may marvel at the fine texture and print of a book as we pursue a research activity necessary to write our report. "I believe it is a mistake," argued Yuriko Saito, "to find aesthetic value in everyday objects and activities only insofar as we momentarily isolate them from their everyday use and contemplate them as if they were art objects created specifically for display. If we divorce them from their practical significance in our lives, we will miss a rich array of aesthetic values integrated with utilitarian contexts."[23]

If using something evokes a genuine aesthetic experience, making something involves no less an aesthetic encounter. (Of course, in making an object, it is always possible to pay no attention to its aesthetic value.) The truth of this claim is confirmed when we make an addition or a modification to our homes. When I decided to erect a picket fence around my yard, I first purchased the posts and the pickets. I took into account the quality of the materials and the estimated size and look of the fence. As I put the posts into the ground and placed the pickets, I kept looking at the results of my work in progress and asked myself: how will it appear? Will the distance between the posts, as well as the height of the pickets, look right? As Roger Scruton pointed out in his inspiring reflections on the aesthetics of everyday life, these questions cannot be answered "in functional or utilitarian terms."[24] My building of the fence, during which I thought about modifications, made comparisons, blended the work of my hands with the judgment of my eyes, was not only an activity undertaken for reaching a practical purpose. It was also an aesthetic endeavour for making something that looked both right and attractive. The criteria I used to install an aesthetically appealing fence were an integral part of the functional choices I made in carrying out the work.

In various areas of our everyday lives – in restaurants, shops, schools, libraries, hospitals, athletic and cultural venues, or in our homes – we may elicit and appreciate simultaneously both the useful and the aesthetic. John Dewey believed that all sorts of professionals value the "completeness of their perceptual experience."[25] They do not want to go along simply with an exclusive commitment to expediency. They aspire to make their actions aesthetically valuable. The execution of their task is smooth and efficient, and also refined, pleasurable to the senses. Nurses and assistants who work in operating rooms often admire the beauty and ease of an operation performed by a skilled surgeon. Students may appreciate the science teacher's imaginative and elegant presentation of theories and experiments.[26]

This insistence on giving equal value to both aesthetic skill and practical purpose may permeate several levels of human life; it may become manifest while conversing with colleagues, delivering a convincing speech, engaging in a professional or volunteer activity, or contributing to the common good.[27] When people free themselves from an undivided focus on useful achievement and are able to imagine how things and actions appear when viewed from different angles and how others perceive them, playfulness in the guise of spontaneous responsiveness, ease, risk, or humour may also become an integral part of their activities. They just need to step courageously beyond the utilitarian standards of the time and place and trust their own judgment about whether the occasion is right, for instance, to let the body's indwelling sense of ease perform a delicate act of repair or restoration, or to bring humour into a community project of planting trees. The perception that allows the emotional aspects of things to come forth freely weans us away from restricted goal-oriented interests, and thus shifts or removes the limits of what can be done and expressed playfully.

The intertwining of practical interest and aesthetic percipience brings satisfaction on another level of our existence. "Civil manners are aesthetically pleasing and morally right," wrote Edward Shils.[28] "Courtesy," as Guardini reminded us, "is a thing of beauty and makes life beautiful. It is 'form': an attitude, gesture, or action which does not merely serve a purpose, but also expresses a meaning which has a value in itself, namely, the dignity of man."[29] There are several other "things of beauty" – politeness, gratitude, selfless and generous giving – that make our everyday societal interactions and surroundings more pleasant, more human. They all imply the recognition of the whole of the person and his or her desire to value both the meaning and the sensuous appearance of a thing or an action and, for a time being, not to attach importance only to its purpose.

There are, indeed, "aesthetic kinds of moral refinement" (Hartmann) that easily lead to the adoption of a play attitude. When we are engaged in a business-related discussion, we tend to start by playfully addressing selected topics, asking questions and listening carefully to what evokes an interest in our interlocutor in a given moment. When we give someone a gift, the choice of the right moment and right words, adapted to the character of the person and his or her circumstances, is often more important to the recipient than the gift itself. Here again, we need to explore playfully the available options before implementing what appears to be the most suitable one. Both forms of human interaction require all sorts of detours, time to linger and delay. Both leave ample room for the playful exploration of formalities. Both involve the virtue of benignity, which is inseparable from our good will, from our willingness to place ourselves in the skin of others, and which is acutely aware of the insufficiency of wanting to make a gift or to reach an agreement. What truly matters is the manner of giving or of negotiating in full respect for the dignity and uniqueness of the person who receives the gift or hears our proposals.

Epilogue

"Why should we value the above-mentioned qualities as well as the various manifestations of the attitude of play?" someone will ask in spirited tone. My reply to this question would likely be to repeat the words of renowned composer and ethnomusicologist Zoltán Kodály. When asked why he attached so much importance to collecting folk songs in remote villages, he responded: "For nothing and for everything ... for the simple reason that life should be lived in its fullness."[1] I might add the winged words of George Santayana: "We may measure the degree of happiness and civilization which any race has attained by the proportion of its energy which is devoted to free and generous pursuits, to the adornment of life and the culture of the imagination. For it is in the spontaneous play of his faculties that man finds himself and his happiness."[2] And further, if this inquiring person were to persist in asking additional questions about the significance of play attitude, I would briefly advance four reasons; these would pertain primarily to the art and value of a truly comprehensive life and less to educational benefits and achievements, and hardly at all to a call to spend more time playing. The educational benefits of a playful attitude are indirect, presenting themselves by implication, when we do not explicitly look for them; as I pointed out earlier, they are possible side effects of activities carried out with a play attitude at home, at school, in a work place, during travel, or in any other context.

In the first place, we find again the delights that our childhood provided in abundance. Ferdinand Ulrich, in his book on the anthropology of childhood, sees in childhood an "existential" of human being which fades away for a while and which, at a certain stage of human life, reasserts itself to mitigate the repressive and debilitating effects of an impersonal and abstract world.[3] Childhood is the symbol of the possibility of beginning something, of remaining flexible and adaptable, and of achieving an original, vivid, and promising perception of living and of solid realities. We relive our childhood on occasions when we enjoy an activity according to its own merits and not merely for the attainment of useful ends, when this activity expresses an unconfined energy and a carefree naïveté, and when we feel the elemental joy of being fully alive and producing something through the free and fearless use of our abilities. Just like the child, we find a joy in digging, making paths, placing interlocking bricks, building gardens, and protecting our plants and trees with decorative fences. We become, once again, lovers of solidity. There are occasions, Vladimir Nabokov tells us, when we retrieve in ourselves the child's "urge to reshape the earth, to act upon a friable environment."[4] We become a child again when we courageously deviate from conventions, cease to behave properly, and create innovative acts of harmless mischief. We return to the habits of our childhood when we prefer the tangible and particular over the abstract and general, when we fearlessly use our common sense and show strong dislike for white lies and hypocrisy, and when we believe, once again, in the aliveness and animation of immanent realities and treat them as images conveying some sort of autonomy and exhibiting an expressive appeal and variability. We, then, live in a responsive world, a world in which we meet things with their desire to play with us. "Children," says Paul Valéry, "grasp in things their useless and real aspects. For nothing is more imaginary than practical perception … They see what is pointless and has no other purpose than to provide an immediate *amusement*, to nourish their imagination without experience, without specialty."[5] It is in this responsive world that playful interactions and unselfish communications occur; we relate to others with confidence, sincerity, and disinterestedness and, at the same time, we readily recognize that, in our encounter with a friend or a colleague, an element of ritual, of charade, and even of light-hearted joking can find its proper place. In short, we recognize ourselves as responsive beings and, notwithstanding the risk of being deceived, this trustful openness and abandonment to the responsive world fills us with contentment.

Learning how to make good use of the free time of our everyday life, and after retirement, how to undertake fulfilling activities, alone or in the company of friends, is not an easy task. Adolf Portmann believed that an "inner attitude of free activity, of the playful life, of meaningfully planned free time" should be adopted early in one's professional life. By doing so, we may avert the frustration and unhappiness of not knowing what to do with the abundance of available leisure time at the twilight of our lives. The disposition that makes this stage of life richer must be formed by our imagination and our awareness of our bodily aptitudes. It preserves the child's capacity for spontaneous inventions and ingenious responsiveness to animated realities and values the joy arising from affective intimacy with the world. Instead of dolls, lego pieces or spinning tops, natural elements – waves, rocks, wind, lawn, snow – become our cherished toys. "No wonder that the playing child is a symbol."[6]

My second reason would be that the adoption of a play attitude allows us to experience our body and its abilities with a feeling of unity. In our everyday life, we tend to view the body as an instrument, a machine, or an object of possession that silently and, ideally, efficiently, deals with tasks and obstacles. We like to think that, in all our sensory-motor experiences, the disembodied mind proposes and the mindless body disposes. In fact, during the process of learning any skill, we entertain this kind of relation to our body. Once a skill is acquired, however, it is possible to give up the habitual desire to observe and control the movements and let our body propose both habitual and unusual responses to the requirements of a situation. In this state, we execute the appropriate movements spontaneously, without thinking about the right technique or calculating the possible outcome of our achievement.

Our bodies often surprise us. All of us notice from time to time that our body can move naturally, without much conscious effort. We might carve a piece of wood or play on a musical instrument without pondering what our hands or feet ought to do. In these moments, as the will to control the body withdraws and the execution of the movement becomes effortless, we experience the pleasant sensation of total involvement and the feeling of harmony and oneness with our body as well as with the different aspects of the motor situation.

Our relationship to the body coincides with our manner of relating to our ambient world. When we experience our body with a sense of unity and of integration, we tend to find our immediate surroundings stimulating and friendly. Conversely, when we perceive concrete and tangible realities as responsive supports for our actions, we also experience our living body with a feeling of unity. We then have the pleasant impression of being carried by our body's indwelling energy and competence.

The quality of successful and complete integration is not easily achieved. For many of us, the task of relaxing our self-consciousness and self-will, on every front and at the same time, is just too difficult. For that reason, we ought to identify in our immediate environment activities that no longer require conscious learning and monitoring, thus making it possible to release ourselves from our habitual objectifying relationship to the world and to ourselves.

When, as we have seen, we adopt an attitude of play, our movements are responsive to the expressive and dynamic structure of things. We enjoy moving with ease, without much exertion. Our pathically tuned body displays its availability and, just as music moves dancing partners, a gesture of tenderness or a beautiful alpine slope elicits a flowing execution of movements. We are, then, able to surrender, without concern or fear, to the abilities of our body – to its natural spontaneity, sensitivity, sense of rhythm, or mimetic aptitude – because we consider a situation not from the point of view of technical efficiency, usefulness, and optimal performance, but from that of meaning, enjoyment, and reciprocity.

Reason number three: by adopting a play attitude we may succeed in transforming our relation to our work activities. One of the central questions steadfastly asked by philosophers, sociologists, educators, and psychologists, and obviously by countless individuals pursuing a professional activity is this: how can work, accomplished under the most diverse conditions – in offices, factories, classrooms, or on agricultural fields, construction sites, and transport vehicles – become a genuinely satisfying, fulfilling experience?

To address this problem, it is worth dwelling briefly on what Giuseppe Rensi has to say, in his recently reissued book, about playful work, which he sees as an integral part of a "fully human life" or of a "spiritual life."[7] What is, then, a spiritual life? Spirit thrives in freedom from constraints, obligations, and duties imposed from without. An activity is spiritual when it asserts its value in itself and is not reduced to the level of a means existing for the sake of an external end, when it expresses a plan, an idea, an image, a feeling – when it is invested with a symbolic content. Work can be spiritual to the extent that it leaves room for the free and creative functioning of the human body. Play activities, indeed any activities undertaken with an attitude of play, are the highest spiritual achievements of human being. Although they may require disciplined preparation and regular practice, such activities are delightful in themselves. While playing or taking up a task with a play attitude, the human spirit evolves in freedom; it enjoys the full and pleasurable concordance of willing and doing, desiring and satisfying obligations, creating symbolic forms and serving a functional purpose.[8]

Rensi believed that the activities of artists, scientists, and philosophers are spiritual activities: they make observations, ask questions, advance hypotheses, propose arguments, initiate research projects, and create forms freely, without being subject to external constraints. Their work is transmuted by passion and genuine fondness, so it is, in fact, "play work." All those who stroll along the streets, engage in a conversation, visit a museum, go to the theatre, attend a concert, hike a mountain, swim in a lake, or simply meditate without any preparation or instruction also carry out, at least for a certain time, "spiritual activities."[9]

Clearly, a truly human life cannot flourish in the absence of a complex and well-functioning social structure, which, for its institution and maintenance, must call for the presence and active contribution of people whose activities are not intrinsically enjoyable. In most areas of our public and private lives, work remains an implacable and often cruel necessity. The so-called spiritual activities draw their sustenance from the tedious and tiresome work accomplished by others, even if, in our time, sophisticated technological devices transform the nature of the fatigue and dreariness.

If unrewarding work remains an inescapable necessity, a daily drudgery, how can we cancel out or at least tone down its negative elements and consequences? Can we accomplish our working tasks without monotony, emptiness, and boredom?

This kind of freedom and playful approach to toiling tasks and activities, Rensi argues, can be enjoyed only in small communities where artisans have workshops and enjoy an unfettered productive existence. They are not bound by the observance of the rules and norms of rigid working conditions. They are still able to carry out their productive activities for no other reason than for the desire to make proficient and pleasurable use of their own capabilities, above all their creative imagination, and thus create well-crafted functional objects – tools, furniture, utensils, potteries, clothing – symbols of their personal feelings and ideas and skills.

Few persons would experience today the "spiritual joy" arising from creative and well-designed artisanal work. Therefore, the question remains to be answered: how can work in our own time become a source of lasting satisfaction? It is clear from the reflections put forward in the previous chapters that a play attitude can be introduced intermittently into all sorts of professional occupations – teaching, diplomacy, health care, trade, commerce, tourism, agriculture, industrial technology, environmental planning and care, public security, engineering, transport, faith-based activities, arts, and other callings. Addressing a problem with humour and ease, responding to and caring about expressive qualities, handling or creating things with an aesthetic sense, and proposing innovative activities in which risks are not minimized remain for many of us today available possibilities in the most diverse practical circumstances. Each of us has to seek occasions that solicit and permit a joyful approach to the task at hand and may change the emotional quality of our milieu even if only for a short time. We can all declare war on pedestrian seriousness, practice cheerfulness, and stop grumbling. We can all quietly rejoice in the intensity of a few memorable moments of our everyday working life and refrain from complaining about their fleeting duration.[10] Providing encouraging and inspiring models to facilitate such a transformation and thus to beautify our lives has been one of the main purposes of this book.

My fourth salient point is this: in an inspiring and fearless educational community, the play attitude in the guise of humour creates a singular atmosphere that is central to the art of teaching. A humorous story is, in my opinion, similar in its compelling sway to a musical piece that we listen to with enchantment. Both are forms of play, both have an intrinsic value and an affective appeal, and both create, beyond the apprehension of their structure and meaning, deeper resonances in us. We are, then, all enticed to follow the unfolding play with our whole being, especially when the melody or the story can sustain our interest by contradicting our expectation and by creating in us a salutary tension. A well-crafted storyline and a captivating musical progression are unpredictable and catch us off guard. The atmosphere of music enhances the spontaneous and playful approach to listening or to performing: we might hum or dance along or perform a piece with relative freedom and inventiveness. Similarly, the atmosphere of humour invites us to involve ourselves in an experience of learning with spontaneity, absorption, and ease. A farce introduced, timely and tactfully, into any kind of teaching activity invigorates our whole being because it appeals not merely to our intellect but also to our belly.[11]

A teaching peppered with humour makes students attentive and awakens what Alfred North Whitehead and others have identified as one of the chief and necessary conditions of any learning: the emotional perception of, and pleasurable interest in, life in all its concrete and abstract manifestations. What is needed is a break introduced into the dreadful monotony of an activity. "The soul cries aloud for release into change ... The transition of humour, wit, irreverence, play, sleep, and – above all – of art are necessary for it."[12] Even the teaching of "serious subjects" such as physics or mathematics would benefit from the sparks ignited by humour, because such sparks would break the dullness of dry facts, provide moments of rest, and dispel the temptation to pedantry. After a quarter of an hour of rote treatment of a subject, an engaging teacher interrupts the flow of the explanation and relates an anecdote, an aphorism, or a humorous illustration invented on the spot. Every student knows that an hour of talk spent with flashes of humour differs in length from an hour of dry lecture. By watching the relaxed and curious faces of students and listening to their pertinent questions, a perceptive teacher notices the value of disciplined teaching interspersed with humorous stories.

There is another strong influence at play in both music and humour. Listening to humorous stories and banter and listening to musical pieces are both communal activities. Sound has the power to draw every listener into its movement and unite them in a collectively shared experience. The sounds and rhythms of a song can create a "community of consonance," to which I have already hinted; they can bring people together and make them hum, dance, walk, or clap the hands together. Time and again participants of family celebrations, sporting events, outdoor concerts, or larger political gatherings observe the uniting power of music. Humour generates a similar experience: it unites people in laughter, makes them feel the energy and elevating power of a group, and grants them the pleasure of togetherness. Gilbert Highet, in his book on the art of teaching, brings to mind the theory of what the French novelist and dramatist Jules Romains called *unanimism*. Unanimism asserts that people remain separate individuals until something – an event, a purpose, an emotion, an institution – joins them into a single collectivity, which, then, starts to feel and think in a way of its own and radiates energy and power. The experience of feeling united with students in the activity of rational thinking, imaginative questioning, wondering, and searching for sanity and certainty gives the greatest pleasure to a teacher and quickens, to the greatest extent, his or her teaching activity with energy and life. This feeling of *syntony* occurs whenever the teacher makes good use of "two powerful instincts which exist in all human beings … *gregariousness* and *the love of play*."[13] And the principal means by which a teacher is able to evoke these instincts and, as a result, to create a "unanimist relationship" with the students is humour. "When a class and its teacher all laugh together, they cease for a time to be separated by individuality, authority, and age. They become a unit, feeling pleasure and enjoying the shared experience."[14] Humour, like music, creates bridges and helps people think and feel in concert. Since the time of learning in the context of apprenticeship, humour has been a central part of teaching on all levels, of proposing riddles, and of celebrating students' achievements. The key to good teaching was then, and is still today, the *shared passion* experienced while laughing and having fun: "Togetherness is the essence of teaching."[15]

Notes

Prologue

1 Lewis, *Four Loves*, 92.
2 Benveniste, "Le jeu comme structure," 161.
3 In his celebrated and much debated book, *Homo Ludens*, Johan Huizinga uses the expressions of play-spirit, play-element, play-quality, play-mood, playfulness when he denotes an attitude, a form of life, or a style of social interaction, presiding over the creative undertakings of eminent individuals or civilizations. This attitude is characterized by diverse physical, moral, aesthetic, and spiritual qualities, among which he singles out spontaneity, elegance, lack of constraint, sense of humour, decency, fair-play, willingness to take risk and face uncertainty, child-like innocence, grandiose carelessness, elasticity of human relationships. The philosopher John Fiske's phrase may be appended to Huizinga's point: "The world's strongest spirits, from Shakespeare down, have been noted for playfulness." "Reminiscences of Huxley," 722.
4 Rubik, *Cubed*, 19.
5 Rombach, *Strukturanthropologie*, 177.
6 Rouet, *André Isoir*, 10.
7 Mumford, *The Urban Prospect*, 28–9.
8 Ibid., 29.
9 Ungar, *Too Safe for Their Own Good*.
10 Rubik calls this constructive approach "playful," which, in his mind, implies an "aura of happiness" and an ability "to see the world for its more positive, even more beautiful side." *Cubed*, 19.
11 Pascal, *Pensées* (Brunschvicg), fragment 139.
12 Henriot, *Le jeu*, 105.
13 Bruner, "Play, Thought, and Language," 69.

14 Several more recent publications have also highlighted the positive contribution of play and playfulness to human existence. Their authors believe that both adults and children enjoy considerable benefit from consciously adopting a more playful approach to life. Here are a few illustrative quotations from scholars, each belonging to a distinct scientific discipline – biology, anthropology, psychology, pedagogy – and each representing a particular cultural milieu – United Kingdom, Siberia and Mongolia, United States, Germany. "The long-term effects of different types of childhood experience remain uncertain. But the overall picture suggests that those who determine the shape of education have much to gain from fostering a positive, playful mood in the learning environment. Playfulness can enhance children's motivation so that they remain interested in a task, rather than getting frustrated and giving up. The adverse consequences of reducing opportunities for physical play and unsupervised social play may include impaired physical fitness, obesity, reduced sociality and reduced creativity." Bateson and Martin, *Play, Playfulness and Innovation*, 21 and 102. "Finally, these Games seem incompatible with the common understanding of the notion: far from being a gratuitous and free amusement, they *had to have* a positive 'effect' on the state of things to come, which is why participation was mandatory. They aimed for action more than distraction. They were not the result of individual initiatives. They expressed a social obligation and a cultural bias." Hamayon, *Why We Play*, 19. "Playing with other children, away from adults, is how children learn to make their own decisions, control their emotions and impulses, see from others' perspectives, negotiate differences with others, and make friends. In short, play is how children learn to take control of their lives." Gray, *Free to Learn*, 157. "Playing is an ability to reckon with unpredictability and to surrender to it. The balance we experience in play between control and serenity, between spoilsport and player, between respecting and challenging the rules, reveals two sides of the art of living." Weiss, "Sich verausgabende Spieler und andere vereinnahmende Falschspieler." 60.

15 Bettelheim, *A Good Enough Parent*, 170.

16 Berger, *The Shape of a Pocket*, 214.

17 Saint-Exupéry, *Terre des hommes*, 197.

18 Plessner, *Laughing and Crying*, 77 and 162. The German translation of Buytendijk's book appeared in 1933 under the title *Wesen und Sinn des Spiels. Das Spielen des Menschen und der Tiere als Erscheinungsform der Lebenstriebe* (Essence and Meaning of Play: The Play of Humans and Animals as Manifestation of Life Drives.)

19 József, "Szerkesztői üzenet" (Message from the Editor), 251. The italics and the translation from Hungarian are mine.

20 Lewis, *The Screwtape Letters*, 53.

21 Chesterton, "Oxford from Without," 63. Similarly, Georges Roditi wanted to see political life freed from the presence of people with dull and dry personalities, devoid of a sense of humour. Humour takes the form "cheerful irony, occasionally turned against oneself." *L'esprit de perfection*, 35.

22 Leroi-Gourhan, *Les Racines du monde*, 181.

23 Ulrich, *Der Mensch als Anfang*, 123.

Chapter One

1 Stevenson, "The Nature of Ethical Disagreement," 1.

2 Lipps, *Die menschliche Natur*, 18–24.

3 Scheler, "Phenomenology and the Theory of Cognition," 137–43.

4 Bollnow, *Einfache Sittlichkeit*, 61.

5 Foucault, "What Is Enlightenment?," 39.

6 See the excellent observations of Thomas De Koninck, "Réflexions sur le bonheur," 149–51.

7 Ulrich, *Der Mensch als Anfang*, 129.

8 Bollnow, *Wesen der Stimmungen*, 154–61.

9 Thomas Aquinas, *Commentary on Aristotle's* De Anima, Book 1, Chapter 8th, 6th Argument.

10 Péguy, *Nous sommes tous à la frontière*, 96–7.

11 Zutt, "Die innere Haltung."

12 Haeffner, *In der Gegenwart leben*, 140–1.

13 Scheler, *On the Eternal in Man*, 265.

14 Hartmann, *Ethics: Volume II*, 306.

15 Ibid., 307.

16 Berger, *Invitation to Sociology*, 98.

17 Buytendijk, "Das Menschliche der menschlichen Bewegung," 181.

18 Murdoch, "Metaphysics and Ethics," 75.

19 Leys, "The Imitation of Our Lord Don Quixote," 28–9.

20 Barzini, *The Italians*, 170.

21 Caillois, *Man, Play, and Games*, 86.

22 Orwell was commissioned to write on the depressed areas of the North of England. On his return to London, he wrote and published *The Road to Wigan Pier*.

23 Mehl, *Attitudes morales*, 5–12.

24 Rothacker, *Geschichtsphilosophie*, 45.

Chapter Two

1 Benveniste, "Le jeu comme structure," 161.

2 Ibid., 166.

3 Seashore, "The Play Impulse and Attitude in Religion," 520.

4 Lewis, *The Four Loves*, 83–4. The Roman Stoic philosopher Seneca held a contrary view when he saw serious philosophy becoming a futile game. *Moral Letters to Lucilius*, 48.

5 Mauriras-Bousquet, "An Appetite for Living," 13. See also her brief analysis of the concept in *Théorie et pratique ludiques*, 25–7. Francine Ferland goes a step further in her well-formulated definition and lists the most important manifestations of the play attitude: "Play is a subjective attitude in which pleasure, curiosity, sense of

humour, and spontaneity are in close relationships; this attitude is reflected in a behaviour that is freely chosen and not tied to the expectation of a specific return." *Modèle ludique*, 34.

6 Highet, "Play and Life," 118.

7 Leroi-Gourhan, *Les Racines du monde*, 166–7.

8 Lorenz, *The Waning of Humaneness*, 66 and 69.

9 Highsmith, *Plotting and Writing Suspense Fiction*, 49. Iris Murdoch emphasized the potential playfulness of the reader when she compared the experience of reading a philosophical text and of immersing oneself in a literary work. "The literary writer deliberately leaves a space for his reader to play in. The philosopher must not leave any space." "Literature and Philosophy," 5.

10 Winnicott, *Playing and Reality*, 44 and 46.

11 Reiners, *Stilkunst*, 313. In German *Einstellung* and *Haltung* are synonyms and I translate both concepts with the English "attitude." *Haltung* emphasizes the lasting and stable characteristic of attitude, while *Einstellung* underscores its dynamic and flexible aspect. According to Jürg Zutt, the difference lies in the ways of taking up an attitude. We adopt (*übernehmen*) a *Haltung* and we gain, acquire (*gewinnen*) an *Einstellung*, as if the initiative was coming from someone or something else. "Die innere Haltung," 33.

12 Kwant, *Phenomenology of Expression*, 84–97.

13 Ibid., 86.

14 Ibid., 96.

15 Sicart, "Playfulness," 21.

16 Ibid., 21.

17 Ibid., 22.

18 Ibid., 26.

19 Lyotard, "Time Today," 73.

20 Alain, *Les idées et les âges*, 119. On the child's earnest sense of obligation, see Henriot, *Existence et obligation*, 235–43. Huizinga's phrase expresses Alain's aphorism in straight prose: "We must emphasize yet again that play does not exclude seriousness." *Homo Ludens*, 180.

21 Riezler, "Play and Seriousness," 506. See also the review of this "valuable discussion" by Ananda K. Coomaraswamy. "We must remember that 'games' ... are not 'merely' physical exercises, spectacles, or amusements, or merely of hygienic or athletic value, but metaphysically significant." "Play and Seriousness," 157.

22 Riezler, "Play and Seriousness," 509.

23 Ibid., 511.

24 Jaspers, *Psychologie der Weltanschauungen*, 49–50.

25 Ibid., 50.

26 Postman, "Amusing Ourselves to Death," 14. See also Postman's book published under the same title: *Amusing Ourselves to Death*, 15–63.

27 Kubey and Csikszentmihalyi, "Television Escape" and "Television Addiction is No Mere Metaphor."

28 Scruton, "Hiding behind the Screen," 104–5.

29 Bateson and Martin, *Play, Playfulness, Creativity and Innovation*, 96. See also Bettelheim, *A Good Enough Parent*, 177–9.

30 Lorenz, *The Waning of Humaneness*, 142–4.

31 Straus, "The Pathology of Compulsion," 321–2.

32 Van Doren, "Joseph and His Brothers," 74.

33 Huxley, "Human Potentialities," 426.

34 Huizinga, *In the Shadow of Tomorrow*, 177–8. Ingeborg Heidemann stressed the same point: "If the world were becoming a play, then, this world would not be for us. Play is only possible when we have the correlate knowledge of non-play." "Philosophische Theorien des Spiels," 321. Roger Caillois also forcefully asserted that the absence of restraint leads to the perversion of play. *Man, Play, and Games*, 44. The reader recalls Jerome Bruner comparing play to a hot house, in which thought, language, and fantasy are combined. He wisely adds a warning: "But do not overheat the hothouse." 69.

35 Huizinga, *Wenn die Waffen schweigen*, III and 169.

36 Gombrich, "Huizinga's *Homo ludens*," 295. "Real civilization," wrote Huizinga, "cannot exist in the absence of a certain play-element, for civilization presupposes limitations and mastery of the self, the ability not to confuse its own tendencies with the ultimate and highest goal, but to understand that it is enclosed within certain bounds freely accepted." *Homo Ludens*, 211.

37 Gombrich, "Huizinga's *Homo ludens*," 295.

38 I borrow the adverb "tragically" from the French writer and former athlete Denis Grozdanovitch, who praises the central elements of the spirit of play – *gratuité*, risk, camaraderie, jubilation over a beautiful gesture, fair-play – in an "age as tragically earnest as our own." "Quelques notes terriblement 'vieux jeu,'" 25.

39 Hammarskjöld, *Markings*, 161.

40 Buytendijk, "Der Spieler," 215.

Chapter Three

1 Buytendijk, "À propos du jeu humain."

2 Bloch, *The Principle of Hope*, 22.

3 Buytendijk, "À propos du jeu humain," 65; Minkowski, "Animer," 246–7.

4 Buytendijk, "Zur Phänomenologie der Begegnung," 73.

5 Gadamer, *Truth and Method*, 105–7.

6 Buytendijk, *Wesen und Sinn des Spiels*, 22–36.

7 In his book on play, Buytendijk acknowledged that he had developed his views on the pathic attitude under the influence of Erwin W. Straus's publications. In his later study on human encounter, however, he correctly distanced himself from Straus's theory, which emphasizes a sharp separation between the pathic and

gnostic relations to things, between sensing and perceiving, between immediate sensory communication with appearances and detached understanding of things with unchanging properties. Indeed, when we first encounter an object, we do not experience it by introducing a clear dividing line between sensing and perceiving, although, at a given moment, one of them may become more prominent. Primarily, we hear a charming melody and not merely tones in sequence; we gaze at the grey clouds lying low over the mountain and portending a storm and not merely at the threatening darkness. See Buytendijk, "Zur Phänomenologie der Begegnung," 69–71. The reader may find Straus's analysis of the pathic communication in his seminal article on lived space, "The Forms of Spatiality," 11–21, and in his book *The Primary World of Senses*, 312–31.

8 Fink, *Grundphänomene des menschlichen Daseins*, 360.

9 Seashore, "The Play Impulse and Attitude in Religion," 520.

10 Langer, *Philosophy in a New Key*, 128. See also the fine observations of Louis Lavelle on the chirping (*pépiement*) of the child. *La parole et l'écriture*, 73–89.

11 Plessner, "Zur Anthropologie der Musik," 190.

12 I borrow this example from Buytendijk's phenomenological analysis of football. *Das Fussballspiel*, 13–14.

13 Langeveld, "Das Ding in der Welt des Kindes," 149–51.

14 Buytendijk, *Das Fussballspiel*, 16.

15 Gadamer, *Truth and Method*, 106.

16 Buytendijk, "Das menschliche Spielen," 113 and 116.

17 Buytendijk, "L'Objectivité des Choses et l'Expressivité des Formes," 427–9.

18 Stevenson, "Child's Play," 135.

19 Tellenbach, "Am Leitfaden des Leibes zu einer anthropologischen Physiologie," 17–18.

20 Marcel, "Leibliche Begegnung," 34–9.

21 Buytendijk, "Some Aspects of Touch," 119–20.

22 Lamb, "The Superannuated Man," 312.

23 Zweig, *Twenty-Four Hours in the Life of a Woman*.

24 Linschoten, "Aspects of Sexual Incarnation."

25 Buytendijk, "Zur Phänomenologie der Begegnung," 95–6.

26 Lewis, *The Four Loves*, 95.

27 Plessner, "On Human Expression," 53–4.

28 Plessner, "Das Lächeln," 432.

29 Lewis, *The Four Loves*, 92.

30 Ibid., 94.

31 Ibid., 92.

32 Ibid., 93.

33 Jünger, *Die Spiele*, 136.

34 Nussbaum, "Sex in the Head," 28.

35 Kwant, *Phenomenology of Expression*, 81.

Chapter Four

1 Schmitz, "Sport and Play," 28.
2 Straus, "The Forms of Spatiality," 21–37.
3 Fink, *Grundphänomene des menschlichen Daseins*, 383.
4 Serres, *Le Tiers-Instruit*, 192.
5 Chesterton, "The Toy Theatre," 108.
6 Arendt and Jaspers, *Correspondence, 1926–1969*, 269.
7 Jean-Paul Sartre sees in this creative act the fundamental trait of play and sport. *L'être et le néant*, 640–7.
8 Welte, "Dasein im Symbol des Spiels," 107–8.
9 Buytendijk, "Unbefangenheit im Umgang."
10 Le Senne, *Obstacle and Value*, 103.
11 Ibid., 102.
12 Minkowski, "Spontaneity," 176.
13 Le Senne, *Obstacle and Value*, 104.
14 Thomas, "Humanities and Science," 150-5. Jacqueline de Romilly proposed a similar approach to her teaching of the structure of Greek sentences. *Écrits sur l'enseignement*, 86-7.
15 Arnheim, "Form and the Consumer," 14.
16 Maugham, *The Summing Up*, 38.
17 James, "The Gospel of Relaxation," 837.
18 Straus, "The Pathology of Compulsion," 314–5.
19 Haeffner, *In der Gegenwart leben*, 163–4.
20 Straus, "The Pathology of Compulsion," 314. Straus translates *Gelassenheit*, used in the original German text, with the English *ease*. I prefer the more comprehensive term *serenity*, which also connotes an activity accomplished with ease.
21 Henriot, *Existence et obligation*, 271–2.
22 Tolstoy, *War and Peace*, 938.
23 Bollnow, *Wesen und Wandel der Tugenden*, 119.
24 Huxley, "Time and the Machine," 123. See also Grozdanovitch, "L'art de se laisser balloter par les circonstances et le courage de laisser faire."
25 Plügge "Über die Arten der menschlichen Befangenheit," 1.
26 Garagorri, "Sur l'esthétique de la conduite."
27 Huxley, *The Human Situation*, 1–11.
28 Ortega y Gasset, "Tierras del Porvenir," 485.
29 Lacoste, *L'idée du beau*, 29.
30 Ibid., 28–30.
31 Rahner, *Man at Play*, 7.

Chapter Five

1 Alain, *Les idées et les âges*, 122.
2 Gadamer, *Truth and Method*, 106.

3   Heckhausen, "Entwurf einer Psychologie des Spielens," 141–2.

4   Haigis, "Das Spiel als Begegnung," 102–13.

5   Kierkegaard, "He Was Believed in the World," 240.

6   Ibid., 245.

7   Huizinga, *Homo Ludens*, 51.

8   Straus, "The Miser," 177.

9   Saint-Exupéry, *Terre des hommes*, 264.

10 Waugh, "Travel – and Escape from Your Friends," 134.

11 Weil, *The Need for Roots*, 32. I have translated the French *jeu* with the English "play" and not with "gamble," which is proposed by the translator of the book.

12 Huizinga, *Homo Ludens*, 203

13 Guttmann, *From Ritual to Record*, 15–55. In a chapter of a recently published book, written in collaboration with Eric Cohen, Leon R. Kass presents a critical account of "adulterated sport" and an outline of sport practised as "artful play," a "gracious display of beautiful form." Their narrative fails, however, to establish a thematic connection between the two guises of sport. *Leading a Worthy Life*, 179–201.

14 Lasch, *Culture of Narcissism*, 102.

15 Chesterton, "The Perfect Game," 21.

16 Schmitz, "Sport and Play," 30–1. In risk sports, Gunnar Breivik tells us, the interaction with certain natural elements gives the activity a playful characteristic. "Climbers are playing with, and on, rock. Sky divers are playing in empty space, with air, and on air pressure. White water kayakers are immersed in running water, in rivers, and are playing with currents, waterfalls, waves and so on." "Dangerous Play with the Elements," 319.

17 Csepregi, *The Clever Body*, 55–61.

18 Buytendijk, *Mensch und Tier*, 67.

19 Simmel, "Flirtation," 134.

20 Ibid., 135.

21 Scheler, "Shame and Feelings of Modesty," 43.

22 Rümke, "Divagations sur le problème," 433.

23 Ibid.

24 Hartmann, "Das Ethos der Persönlichkeit," 663–4.

25 Maldiney, *Penser l'homme et la folie*, 404. For a more thorough study of the subject, see my article "Le problème du temps vécu dans *Le Château de Barbe-Bleue* de Béla Bartók."

26 Caillois, *Man, Play, and Games*, 23–6, 81–97, 132–42.

27 Caillois, *Le fleuve Alphée*, 44.

28 Pessoa, "Three Prose Fragments," 12.

29 Caillois, *Le fleuve Alphée*, 45.

30 Lavelle, *The Dilemma of Narcissus*, 112. I have translated the French *vocation* with the English "calling" and not with "destiny," which is used by the translator of the book.

31 Lasch, *Culture of Narcissism*, 11.

Chapter Six

1 Buytendijk, "À propos du jeu humain," 63–4.

2 Rombach, *Strukturanthropologie*, 176.

3 Nicolson, "The English Sense of Humour," 19.

4 Ibid., 26.

5 Mikes, *English Humour for Beginners*, 32. Mikes's assertion brings to mind the watchword of phenomenology: Back to the things themselves. This rule requires one to focus first on what is given, to respect it as it appears in its complexity and richness, and to exclude, or at least to put aside for a while, theories and traditions. By approaching phenomena in the light of theories, one risks simplifying the complex, curtailing the richness.

6 Rombach, *Strukturanthropologie*, 175.

7 Chesterton, "The Romance of Rostand," 72.

8 Chesterton, "Cockneys and Their Jokes," 17.

9 Chesterton, "Humour," 25.

10 Chesterton, *Autobiography of G.K. Chesterton*, 49.

11 Hartmann, *Aesthetics*, 482.

12 Nicolson, "The English Sense of Humour," 35.

13 Mikes, *English Humour for Beginners*, 70.

14 Frye, "Literature as Therapy," 31.

15 Mikes recounts this "joke of jokes" in his *Humour in Memoriam*, 115. It goes like this: "A Jew goes to the Rabbi in despair and tells him that his son wants to get baptized – regarded as the worst of all blows. 'Well,' says the Rabbi, 'look at my own son.' 'What do you mean?' asks the Jew astonished. 'You do not mean that your own son, Rabbi, wants to get baptized?' 'Yes, that is exactly what I do mean?' 'And what did you do when you heard this?' 'What can a Rabbi do? I turned to God.' 'And what did God tell you?' 'Exactly what I have told you: look at my own son.'"

16 Ritter, "Über das Lachen," 76–84.

17 Idid., 90–1. See also Helga Nowotny's book *The Orderly Messiness*, on playfulness, messiness, and the creative exploration of the world.

18 Knox, "Towards a Philosophy of Humour," 543–6.

19 Auden, "The Joker of the Pack," 255.

20 Serres, *Morales espiègles*, 15–20.

21 Bergson, *Le rire*, 15.

22 Wittgenstein, *Culture and Value*, 83.

23 Thomas De Koninck sees in humour one of the highest manifestations of intelligence. "Qu'est-ce que l'intelligence humaine?," 91–4.

24 Koestler, *Janus*, 109–30.

25 Nussbaum, "Human Functioning and Social Justice," 219.

26 Lersch, "Die Philosophie des Humors," 36.

27 Leroi-Gourhan, *Les Racines du monde*, 181.

28 Neumann, "Über das Lachen," 28.

29 Havel, *Interrogatoire à distance*, 102. Odo Marquard's understanding of the comic throws light on a similar contrast: "The comic produces laughter by making visible the futile in the officially important and the important in the officially futile." Humour throws overboard our standard value judgments. As we have seen, humour stems from an inclination to take everything differently. "Exile der Heiterkeit," 54.

30 Radermacher, *Weinen und Lachen*, 78.

31 Rahner, *Man at Play*, 35–59.

32 Curtius, "Jest and Earnest in Medieval Literature."

33 Tellenbach, "La réalité, le comique et l'humour," 17–18.

34 Mikes, *Humour in Memoriam*, 13.

35 Ibid., 20.

36 Chesterton, "Humour," 23.

37 Ibid., 24.

38 Hartmann, *Aesthetics*, 451.

39 Ibid.

40 Ruch, "Components of Sense of Humor."

41 Nicolson, "The English Sense of Humour," 47.

42 Hartmann, *Aesthetics*, 465–6.

43 Scruton, *Culture Counts*, 45.

44 King, *With Silent Friends*, 82.

45 Haecker, "Über Humor und Satire," 79.

46 Scruton, *Culture Counts*, 48.

Chapter Seven

1 Benveniste, "Le jeu comme structure," 166.

2 Buytendijk, "Der Spieler," 210–13; Portmann, "What Does the Living Form Mean to Us?"

3 Ibid., 211.

4 Guardini, *Vom Geist der Liturgie*; Über das Wesen des Kunstwerks.

5 Guardini, *Vom Geist der Liturgie*, 92.

6 Ibid., 99.

7 A separation between the two forms of attitude does not cancel out the possibility of bringing them together. We may assume a playful mood while undertaking a strictly utilitarian task. We may, for example, introduce some playfulness into the preparation of our yearly budget by attributing to each number a particular pitch of vocal sound. We may then sing playfully our budget. Analyzing this kind of experience, however, is not the subject of this chapter.

8 Scruton, *I Drink Therefore I am*, 195–7. In fact, my translation of Hamvas's essay appeared in 2003, six years before Scruton published his entertaining book. It was reprinted in 2013. Peter Sherwood's new translation was published in 2016. Scruton praised Hamvas's book and related it to his own reflections on drinking wine in an article entitled *Wine and Philosophy*, published in 2010 in the magazine *Decanter*.

9 Hamvas, *The Philosophy of Wine*, 75.

10 Ibid., 52–3.

11 Scruton, *I Drink Therefore I Am*, 159–60.

12 Hamvas, *The Philosophy of Wine*, 48.

13 Sansot, *Du bon usage de la lenteur*, 111.

14 Hamvas, *The Philosophy of Wine*, 88.

15 Sansot, *Du bon usage de la lenteur*, 33.

16 For an overview of published views on the act of strolling in a city, see Borisenkova, "Le flâneur comme lecteur de la ville contemporaine."

17 Buytendijk, *Allgemeine Theorie der menschlichen Haltung und Bewegung*, 297.

18 Worsley, *Shackleton's Boat Journey*, 136.

19 Spaemann, *Basic Moral Concepts*, 76.

20 Dewitte, "Le sens ontologique de l'ornement."

21 Guardini, "Courtesy," 135–7.

22 Ibid., 132.

23 Plessner, *Grenzen der Gemeinschaft*, 111.

24 Ibid., 109, 112.

25 Rensi, *Lettres spirituelles d'un philosophe sceptique*, 18. The italics are mine.

26 James, "The Gospel of Relaxation," 833.

27 Cane, *The Artist in Each of Us*, 21–9.

28 Barzun, "The Indispensable Amateur," 37.

29 Leys "The Prince de Ligne, or the Eighteenth Century Incarnate," 57.

30 Ibid. See also the fine tribute to the amateur in Leys's lecture on Chesterton, 103–5, and in Rubik's book *Cubed: The Puzzle of Us All*, 36–8.

Chapter Eight

1 Alain, *Système des beaux-arts*, 264.

2 Havel, "Politics, Morality, and Civility," 10–12.

3 Hartmann, *Aesthetics*, 466.

4 Benveniste, "Le jeu comme structure," 166.

5 Marcel, "Reply to Otto Friedrich Bollnow," 201; see also Bollnow, "Marcel's Concept of Availability" and Marcel, "Phenomenological Notes on Being in a Situation."

6 Arnheim, "Art among the Objects," 13.

7 Cane, *The Artist in Each of Us*, 22.

8 Ibid.

9 For a more detailed account of the views of these influential scholars, see my book *The Clever Body*.

10 Minkowski, "Spontaneity," 177.

11 Jankélévitch, *Liszt et la rhapsodie*, 91.

12 Helga Nowotny believed that adopting a play attitude is one of the possible ways of facing the "enormous complexity, uncertainty and contingency" of the future. See

her concluding statement made at the Aboagora Symposium in Finland: "Dare to Know, Dare to Tell, Dare to Play," 52–3.

13 Linschoten, "Over de Humor," 655.

14 Hartmann, *Aesthetics*, 465–7.

15 Ibid., 467.

16 Lavelle, The *Dilemma of Narcissus*, 98.

17 Ibid., 100.

18 Mauriras-Bousquet, "An Appetite for Living," 17.

19 Mead, "The Nature of Aesthetic Experience," 297.

20 Cassirer, *An Essay on Man*, 150–2.

21 Hartmann, *Aesthetics*, 58.

22 Geiger, *The Significance of Art*, 195.

23 Saito, *Everyday Aesthetics*, 27.

24 Scruton, *Beauty*, 69.

25 Dewey, *Art as Experience*, 262.

26 John Dewey observed that "compartmentalized psychology" keeps promoting the strict separation of utilitarian and aesthetic interests. Some individuals contend that the disconnection is a reflection of the social tendency to oppose objects envisaged for practical purposes and things offering an aesthetic experience. Others assert that the separation is an essential aspect of our human make-up. "It has been urged that there is an antithesis in the very structure of our being between the fluent action of practice and the vivid consciousness of esthetic experience." Ibid., 261.

27 In her moving book, Marwa Al-Sabouni underscored the value of hand-produced things for the collective effort of creating flourishing and self-sustaining communities in war-torn Syria. The social importance of craft production, which involves the artisan's skills and "special sense of decorum," resides in lifting useful products "into a world of meaning" that a community risks losing in a "totally mechanized age." *The Battle for Home*, 97–9. Years before the publication of this book, Susanne Langer also pleaded in favour of the satisfaction of the worker's "impulse toward symbolic formulation" and desire to find "natural means for expressing the unity of personal life." *Philosophy in a New Key*, 292–3.

28 Shils, "The Virtue of Civility," 339.

29 Guardini, *Learning the Virtues*, 135.

Epilogue

1 Kodály, "Mit akarok a régi székely dalokkal? (What Do I Want to Do with the Old Sekler Songs?)," 29.

2 Santayana, *The Sense of Beauty*, 18–19.

3 Ulrich, *Der Mensch als Anfang*, 125.

4 Nabokov, *Speak, Memory*, 302. Similarly, Molly Brearley correctly asserted that the "basic pleasure in 'being a cause'" permeates children's earliest contact with the material world. "Play in Childhood," 322.

5 Valéry, "Mélange," 397.

6 Portmann, "Spiel und Leben," 249–50.

7 Rensi, *Contre le travail*, 71. Published in 2017, this French translation is from the middle part of Rensi's larger book entitled *L'Irrazionale, Il lavoro, L'amore*.

8 See also Langer, *Philosophy in a New Key*, 289–94.

9 Rensi, *Contre le travail*, 24–42.

10 Forster, "The Beauty of Life," 172.

11 Maugham, *Selected Prefaces and Introductions of W. Somerset Maugham*, 41.

12 Whitehead, *Science and the Modern World*, 234.

13 Highet, *The Art of Teaching*, 63.

14 Ibid. In their recently published book, Maggie Berg and Barbara K. Seeber also argued that humour and laughter promote "social harmony" in the classroom. *The Slow Professor*, 44–5.

15 Highet, *The Art of Teaching*, 64.

Bibliography

Alain, *Les idées et les âges*. In *Les Passions et la Sagesse*, 1–321. Paris: Gallimard, Bibliothèque de la Pléiade, 1994.

– *Système des beaux-arts*. In *Les arts et les dieux*, 215–467. Paris: Gallimard, Bibliothèque de la Pléiade, 1968.

Al-Sabouni, Marwa. *The Battle for Home: The Vision of a Young Architect in Syria*. New York: Thames & Hudson Inc., 2016.

Arendt, Hannah, and Karl Jaspers. *Correspondence, 1926–1969*. Edited by Lotte Köhler and Hans Saner, translated by Robert Kimber and Rita Kimber. New York: Harcourt, Brace, Jovanovich, 1992.

Arnheim, Rudolf. "Art among the Objects." In *To the Rescue of Arts: Twenty–Six Essays*, 7–14. Berkeley: University of California Press, 1992.

– "Form and the Consumer." In *Toward a Psychology of Art: Collected Essays*, 7–16. Berkeley: University of California Press, 1972.

Auden, W.H. "The Joker in the Pack." In *The Dyer's Hand and Other Essays*, 246–72. New York: Random House, 1962.

Barzini, Luigi. *The Italians: A Full-Length Portrait Featuring Their Manners and Morals*. New York: Touchstone, 1996.

Barzun, Jacques. "The Indispensable Amateur." In *Critical Questions: On Music and Letters, Culture and Biography, 1940–1980*, selected, edited, and introduced by Bea Friedland, 30–8. Chicago: University of Chicago Press, 1982.

Bateson, Patrick, and Paul Martin. *Play, Playfulness, Creativity and Innovation*. Cambridge: Cambridge University Press, 2013.

Benveniste, Émile. "Le jeu comme structure." *Deucalion* 2 (1947): 161–7.

Berg, Maggie, and Barbara K. Seeber. *The Slow Professor: Challenging the Culture of Speed in the Academy*. Toronto: University of Toronto Press, 2016.

Berger, John. *The Shape of a Pocket*. New York: Pantheon Books, 2001.

Berger, Peter L. *Invitation to Sociology: A Humanistic Perspective.* Garden City, New York: Anchor Books, 1963.

Bergson, Henri. *Le rire. Essai sur la signification du comique.* Paris: Presses universitaires de France, 1985.

Bettelheim, Bruno. *A Good Enough Parent: A Book on Child-Rearing.* New York: Vintage Books, 1988.

Bloch, Ernst. *The Principle of Hope: Volume 1.* Translated by Neville Plaice, Stephen Plaice, and Paul Knight. Cambridge: MIT PRESS, 1995.

Bollnow, Otto Friedrich. *Einfache Sittlichkeit. Schriften Band III.* Würzburg: Könighausen & Neumann, 2009.

– "Marcel's Concept of Availability." In *The Philosophy of Gabriel Marcel,* edited by Paul Arthur Schilpp and Lewis Edwin Hahn, 177–99. La Salle, Illinois: Open Court Publishing, 1984.

– *Wesen der Stimmungen.* 5th ed. Frankfurt am Main: Verlag Vittorio Klostermann, 1974.

– *Wesen und Wandel der Tugenden.* Frankfurt am Main: Ullstein Verlag, 1981.

Borisenkova, Anna. "Le flâneur comme lecteur de la ville contemporaine." *Russian Sociological Review* 16, no. 2 (2017): 75–88.

Brearley, Molly. "Play in Childhood." *Philosophical Transactions of the Royal Society of London.* Series B, Biological Sciences, volume 251, no. 772 (1966): 321–5.

Breivik, Gunnar. "Dangerous Play with the Elements: Towards a Phenomenology of Risk Sports." *Sport, Ethics and Philosophy* 5 (2011): 314–30.

Bruner, Jerome. "Play, Thought, and Language." *Peabody Journal of Education* 60, no. 3 (1983): 60–9.

Buytendijk, F.J.J. *Allgemeine Theorie der menschlichen Haltung und Bewegung.* Berlin: Springer-Verlag, 1956.

– *Das Fussballspiel. Eine psychologische Studie.* Würzburg: Werkbund Verlag, 1953.

– *Mensch und Tier. Ein Beitrag zur vergleichenden Psychologie.* Reinbek: Rowohlt, 1958.

– "Das Menschliche der menschlichen Bewegung." In *Das Menschliche. Wege zu seinem Verständnis,* 208–40. Stuttgart: Koehler Verlag, 1958.

– "Das menschliche Spielen." In *Kulturanthropologie,* edited by Hans–Georg Gadamer and Paul Vogler, 88–122. Stuttgart: Deutscher Taschenbuch Verlag, 1973.

– "L'Objectivité des Choses et l'Expressivité des Formes." *Psychiatria, Neurologia, Neurochirurgica* 73 (1970): 427–31.

– "Zur Phänomenologie der Begegnung." In *Das Menschliche. Wege zu seinem Verständnis,* 60–100. Stuttgart: Koehler Verlag, 1958.

– "À propos du jeu humain." *L'évolution psychiatrique* 1956 (1): 63–7.

– "Some Aspects of Touch." *Journal of Phenomenological Psychology* 1 (1970): 99–124.

– "Der Spieler." In *Das Menschliche. Wege zu seinem Verständnis,* 170–88. Stuttgart: Koehler Verlag, 1958.

– "Unbefangenheit im Umgang." In Frederik J.J. Buytendijk, Martinus Jan Langeveld, and Antoon Vergote, *Unbefangen sein als Weg zur Selbstverwirklichung,* 9–33. Köln: J.P. Bachem Verlag, 1973.

– *Wesen und Sinn des Spiels. Das Spielen des Menschen und der Tiere als Erscheinungsform der Lebenstriebe* (1933). Reprint ed. New York: Arno Press, 1976.

Caillois, Roger. *Le fleuve Alphée*. Paris: Gallimard, 1978.

– *Man, Play, and Games*. Translated by Meyer Barash. Urbana and Chicago: University of Illinois Press, 2001.

Cane, Florence. *The Artist in Each of Us*. Revised ed. Crafstbury Common, Vermont: Art Therapy Publications, 1983.

Cassirer, Ernst. *An Essay on Man: An Introduction to a Philosophy of Human Culture*. New Haven: Yale University of Press, 2021.

Chesterton, G.K. *The Autobiography of G.K. Chesterton*. San Francisco: Ignatius Press, 2006.

– "Cockneys and their Jokes." In *All Things Considered*, 9th ed., 13–20. London: Methuen, 1915.

– "Humour." In *The Spice of Life*, 22–9. Chester Springs, Pennsylvania: Dufour Editions, 1966.

– "Oxford from Without." In *All Things Considered*, 9th ed., 60–6. London: Methuen, 1915.

– "The Perfect Game." In *Tremendous Trifles*, 19–22. Auckland: Floating Press, 2009.

– "The Romance of Rostand." In *The Uses of Diversity: A Book of Essays*, 71–4. London: Methuen, 1921.

– "The Toy Theatre." In *Tremendous Trifles*, 105–9. Auckland: Floating Press, 2009.

Coomaraswamy, Ananda K. "Play and Seriousness." In *Selected Papers. Volume 2: Metaphysics*, edited by Roger Lipsey, 156–8. Princeton: Princeton University Press, 1987.

Csepregi, Gabor. *The Clever Body*. Calgary: University of Calgary Press, 2006.

– "Le problème du temps vécu dans *Le Château de Barbe-Bleue* de Béla Bartók." *Revue Musicale de Suisse Romande* 58, 3 (2005): 28–37.

Curtius, E.R. "Jest and Earnest in Medieval Literature." In *European Literature and the Latin Middle Ages*, translated by Willard R. Trask, 417–35. London: Routledge & Kegan Paul, 1953.

De Koninck, Thomas. "Qu'est-ce que l'intelligence humaine?" In *Questions ultimes*, 53–110. Ottawa: Presses de l'Université d'Ottawa, 2012.

– "Réflexions sur le bonheur." In *Questions ultimes*, 137–72. Ottawa: Presses de l'Université d'Ottawa, 2012.

Dewey, John. *Art as Experience*. New York: Perigee Books, 1980.

Dewitte, Jacques. "Le sens ontologique de l'ornement." In *La manifestation de soi. Éléments d'une critique philosophique de l'utilitarisme*, 64–81. Paris: La Découverte, 2010.

Ferland, Francine. *Le modèle ludique. Le jeu, l'enfant ayant une déficience physique et l'ergothérapie*. Montreal: Presses de l'Université de Montréal, 2003.

Fink, Eugen. *Grundphänomene des menschlichen Daseins*. Edited by Egon Schütz and Franz-Anton Schwarz. Freiburg: Verlag Karl Alber, 1979.

Fiske, John. "Reminiscences of Huxley." In *Annual Report of the Board of Regents of the Smithsonian Institution*. Washington: Government Printing Office, 1901, 713–28.

Forster, E.M. "The Beauty of Life." In *Albergo Empedocle and Other Writings*, edited by George H. Thomson, 169–75. New York: Liveright, 1971.

Foucault, Michel. "What Is Enlightenment?" In *The Foucault Reader*, edited by Paul Rabinow, 32–50. New York: Pantheon Books, 1984.

Frye, Northrop. "Literature as Therapy." In *The Eternal Act of Creation: Essays, 1979–1990*, edited by Robert D. Denham, 21–34. Bloomington & Indianapolis: Indiana University Press, 1993.

Gadamer, Hans-Georg. *Truth and Method*. Second revised ed. Translation revised by Joel Weinsheimer and Donald G. Marshall. London: Continuum, 2006.

Garagorri, Paulino. "Sur l'esthétique de la conduite." *Revue de Métaphysique et de Morale* 66 (1961): 136–41.

Geiger, Moritz. *The Significance of Arts: A Phenomenological Approach to Aesthetics*. Edited and translated by Klaus Berger. Washington, D.C.: Center for Advanced Research in Phenomenology & University Press of America, 1986.

Gombrich, E.H. "Huizinga's *Homo ludens*." In *Johan Huizinga 1872–1972: Papers Delivered to the Johan Huizinga Conference Groningen 11–15 December 1972*, edited by W.R.H. Koops, E.H. Kossmann, and G. van der Plaat, 133–54. The Hague: Martinus Nijhoff, 1973.

Gray, Peter. *Free to Learn: Why Unleashing the Instinct to Play Will Make Our Children Happier, More Self-Reliant, and Better Students for Life*. New York: Basic Books, 2013.

Grozdanovitch, Denis. "L'art de se laisser balloter par les circonstances et le courage de laisser faire." In *L'art difficile de ne presque rien faire*, 162–8. Paris: Denoël, 2009.

– "Quelques notes terriblement 'vieux jeu.'" *Revue du Mauss*. 45 (2015, no. 1): 25–43.

Guardini, Romano. "Courtesy." In *Learning the Virtues that Lead You to God*, translated by Stella Lange, 129–40. Manchester, New Hampshire: Sophia Institute Press, 2013.

– *Vom Geist der Liturgie*. Freiburg im Breisgau: Verlag Herder, 1983.

– *Über das Wesen des Kunstwerks*. Mainz: Matthias-Grünewald Verlag, 2005.

Guttmann, Allen. *From Ritual to Record: The Nature of Modern Sports*. Updated, with a new afterword. New York: Columbia University Press, 2004.

Haecker, Theodor. "Über Humor und Satire." In *Dialog über Christentum und Kultur, mit einem Exkurs über Sprache, Humor und Satire*, 73–95. Hellerau: Verlag Jakob Hegner, 1930.

Haeffner, Gerd. *In der Gegenwart leben. Auf der Spur eines Urphänomens*. Stuttgart: Verlag W. Kohlhammer, 1996.

Haigis, Ernst. "Das Spiel als Begegnung. Versuch einer materialen Spieldeutung." *Zeitschrift für Psychologie*. Band 150, Heft 1, 92–167. Nachdruck 1968. Leipzig: Johann Ambrosius Barth Verlag, 1941.

Hamayon, Roberte. *Why We Play: An Anthropological Study*. Translated by Damien Simon. Chicago: Hau Books, 2016.

Hammarskjöld, Dag. *Markings*. Translated by Leif Sjöberg and W.H. Auden. New York: Alfred A. Knopf, 1965.

Hamvas, Béla. *The Philosophy of Wine*. Translated by Gabor Csepregi. Szentendre: Editio M, 2013.

Hartmann, Nicolai. *Aesthetics*. Translated by Eugene Kelly. Berlin/Boston: Walter de Gruyter GmbH, 2014.

– *Ethics. Volume 1: Moral Phenomena*. Translated by Stanton Coit. London: George Allen and Unwin, 1932.

– *Ethics. Volume 2: Moral Values*. Translated by Stanton Coit. Atlantic Highlands, New Jersey: Humanities Press 1963.

– "Das Ethos der Persönlichkeit." *Neue Schweizer Rundschau* 18 (1950–51): 657–64.

Havel, Vaclav. *Interrogatoire à distance. Entretien avec Karel Hvizd'ala*. Translated by Jan Rubes. La Tour d'Aigues: Éditions de l'Aube, 1989.

– "Politics, Morality, and Civility." In *Summer Meditations*, translated by Paul Wilson, 1–20. Toronto: Alfred A. Knopf Canada, 1992.

Heckhausen, Heinz. "Entwurf einer Psychologie des Spielens." In *Das Kinderspiel*, edited by Andreas Flitner, 138–55. Munich: Piper Verlag, 1978.

Heidemann, Ingeborg. "Philosophische Theorien des Spiels." *Kant-Studien* 50 (1959): 316–22.

Henriot, Jacques. *Existence et obligation*. Paris: Presses universitaires de France, 1967.

– *Le jeu*. Paris: Presses universitaires de France, 1969.

Highet, Gilbert. "Play and Life." In *Explorations*, 117–19. New York: Oxford University Press, 1971.

– *The Art of Teaching*. New York: Alfred A. Knopf, 1951.

Highsmith, Patricia. *Plotting and Writing Suspense Fiction*. New York: St. Martin's Griffin, 1983.

Huizinga, Johan. *Homo Ludens: A Study of the Play-Element in Culture*. Boston: Beacon Press, 1955.

– *In the Shadow of Tomorrow*. Translated by J.H. Huizinga. New York: W.W. Norton, 1964.

– *Wenn die Waffen schweigen. Die Aussichten auf Genesung unserer Kultur*. Translated by Wolfgang Hirsch. Basel: Burg-Verlag, 1945.

Huxley, Aldous. "Human Potentialities." In *The Humanist Frame*, edited by Julian Huxley, 417–32. Freeport, New York: Books for Libraries Press, 1972.

– *The Human Situation: Lectures at Santa Barbara, 1959*. Edited by Piero Ferrucci. London: Flamingo Modern Classic, 1994.

– "Time and the Machine." In *The Olive Tree*, 122–4. London: Chatto & Windus, 1947.

James, William. "The Gospel of Relaxation." In *Writings 1878-1899*, edited by Gerald Myers, 825–40. New York: Library of America, 1992.

Jankélévitch, Vladimir. *Liszt et la rhapsodie. Essai sur la virtuosité*. Paris: Plon, 1989.

Jaspers, Karl. *Psychologische der Weltanschauungen*. Berlin: Verlag von Julius Springer, 1919.

József, Attila. "Szerkesztői üzenet" (Message from the Editor). In *Tanulmányok, cikkek, levelek* (Studies, Articles, Letters), 248–52. Budapest: Szépirodalmi Könykiadó, 1977.

Jünger, Friedrich Georg. *Die Spiele. Ein Schlüssel zu Ihrer Bedeutung*. Frankfurt am Main: Verlag Vittorio Klostermann, 1953.

Kass, Leon R. *Leading a Worthy Life: Finding Meaning in Modern Times*. New York: Encounter Books, 2017.

Kierkegaard, Søren. "He Was Believed in the World." In *Christian Discourses*, edited and translated by Howard V. Hong and Edna Hong, 234–46. Princeton, New Jersey: Princeton University Press, 1997.

King, Richard. *With Silent Friends*. London: Bodley Head Ltd., 1933.

Knox, Israel. "Towards a Philosophy of Humour." *The Journal of Philosophy* 47 (1951): 541–8.

Kodály, Zoltán. "Mit akarok a régi székely dalokkal? (What Do I Want with the Old Sekler Songs?)." In *Visszatekintés* (Looking Back), vol. 1, edited by Ferenc Bónis, 29–30. Budapest: Editio Musica, 1989.

Koestler, Arthur. *Janus: A Summing Up*. New York: Random House, 1978.

Kubey, Robert, and Mihaly Csikszentmihalyi. "Television Addiction is No Mere Metaphor." *Scientific American* 286, 2 (February 2002): 74–80.

– "Television as Escape: Subjective Experience Before an Evening of Heavy Viewing." In Mihaly Csikszentmihalyi, *Flow and the Foundations of Positive Psychology: The Collected Works of Mihaly Csikszentmihalyi*. 103–11. Dordrecht: Springer-Verlag, 2014.

Kwant, Remy C. *Phenomenology of Expression*. Pittsburgh: Duquesne University Press, 1969.

Lacoste, Jean. *L'idée de beau*. Paris: Presses universitaires de France, 1981.

Lamb, Charles. "The Superannuated Man." In *The Portable Charles Lamb*, edited by John Mason Brown, 306–15. New York: Viking Press, 1964.

Langer, Susanne K. *Philosophy in a New Key: A Study in the Symbolism of Reason, Rite, and Art*. 3rd ed. Cambridge, Massachusetts: Harvard University Press, 1957.

Langeveld, Martinus J. "Das Ding in der Welt des Kindes." In *Studien zur Anthropologie des Kindes*. 2nd enlarged ed., Erweiterte Auflage, 142–56. Tübingen: Max Niemeyer, 1964.

Lasch, Christopher. *Culture of Narcissism: American Life in an Age of Diminishing Expectations*. New York: W.W. Norton, 1978.

Lavelle, Louis. *The Dilemma of Narcissus*. Translated by W.T. Gairdner. London: George Allen & Unwin Ltd, 1973.

– *La parole et l'écriture*. Paris: L'artisan du livre, 1947.

Leroi-Gourhan, André. *Les Racines du monde. Entretiens avec Claude-Henri Rocquet*. Paris: Pierre Belfond, 1982.

Lersch, Philipp. "Die Philosophie des Humors." In *Der Mensch als Schnittpunkt. Fragen zur Psychologie und Anthropologie der Gegenwart*, 172–6. München: Verlag C.H. Beck, 1969.

Le Senne, René. *Obstacle and Value*. Translated by Bernard P. Dauenhauer. Evanston: Northwestern University Press, 1972.

Lewis, C.S. *Four Loves*. London: Fount Paperbacks, 1981.

– *The Screwtape Letters*. New York: HarperCollins, 2015.

Leys, Simon. "Chesterton: The Poet Who Dances With a Hundred Legs." In *The Hall of Uselessness: Collected Essays*. 100–13. New York: New York Review of Books, 2013.

– "The Imitation of Our Lord Don Quixote." In *The Hall of Uselessness: Collected Essays*. 17–30. New York: New York Review of Books, 2013.

– "The Prince de Ligne, or the Eighteenth Century Incarnate." In *The Hall of Uselessness: Collected Essays*. 55–60. New York: New York Review of Books, 2013.

Linschoten, Jan. "Aspects of the Sexual Incarnation: An Inquiry Concerning the Meaning of the Body in Sexual Encounter." In *Phenomenological Psychology: The Dutch School*, edited by Joseph J. Kockelmans, 149–94. Dordrecht: Martinus Nijhoff, 1987.

– "Over de Humor." *Tijdschrift voor Philosophie* 13 (1951): 603–66.

Lipps, Hans. *Die menschliche Natur.* 2nd ed. Frankfurt am Main: Verlag Vittorio Klostermann, 1977.

Lorenz, Konrad. *The Waning of Humaneness.* Translated by Robert Warren Kickert. Boston: Little, Brown and Company, 1987.

Lyotard, Jean-François. "Time Today." In *The Inhuman: Reflections on Time*, translated by Bennington, Geoffrey, and Rachel Bowlby, 58–77. Stanford: Stanford University Press, 1991.

Maldiney, Henri. *Penser l'homme et la folie. À la lumière de l'analyse existentielle et de l'analyse du destin.* Grenoble: Jérôme Millon, 1991.

Marcel, Gabriel. "Leibliche Begegnung. Notizen aus einem gemeinsamen Gedankengang." In *Leiblichkeit. Philosophische, gesellschaftliche und therapeutische Perspektiven*, edited by Hilarion Petzold, 15–46. Padeborn: Junfermann-Verlag, 1986.

– "Phenomenological Notes on Being in a Situation." In *Creative Fidelity*, translated by Robert Rosthal, 82–103. New York: Fordham University Press, 2002.

– "Reply to Otto Friedrich Bollnow." In *The Philosophy of Gabriel Marcel*, edited by Paul Arthur Schilpp and Lewis Edwin Hahn, 200–3. La Salle, Illinois: Open Cour Publishing Company, 1984.

Marquard, Odo. "Exile der Heiterkeit." In *Aesthetica und Anaesthetica. Philosophische Überlegungen*, 47–63. Paderborn: Verlag Ferdinand Schöningh, 1989.

Maugham, W. Somerset. *Selected Prefaces and Introductions of W. Somerset Maugham.* London: Heinemann, 1963.

– *The Summing Up.* New York: The Literary Guild of America, Inc., 1938.

Mauriras-Bousquet. Martine. "*An Appetite for Living.*" The UNESCO *Courier* (MAY 1991): 13–17.

– *Théorie et pratique ludiques.* Paris: Economica, 1984.

Mead, H. George. "The Nature of Aesthetic Experience." In *Selected Writings*, edited by Andrew J. Reck, 294–305. Indianapolis: Bobbs-Merrill, 1964.

Mehl, Roger. *Les attitudes morales.* Paris: Presses universitaires de France, 1971.

Mikes, George. *English Humour for Beginners.* London: Andre Deutsch, 1980.

– *Humour in Memoriam.* London: Routledge & Kegan Paul, 1970.

Minkowski, Eugène. "Animer." In *Vers une cosmologie. Fragments philosophiques*, 246–58. Paris: Aubier-Montaigne, 1967.

– "Spontaneity (…Spontaneous Movement Like this!)." In *Readings in Existential Phenomenology*, edited by Nathaniel Lawrence and Daniel O'Connor, 168–77. Englewood: Prentice-Hall, 1967.

Mumford, Lewis. *The Urban Prospect.* New York: Harcourt, Brace & World, Inc., 1968.

Murdoch, Iris. "Literature and Philosophy: A Conversation with Bryan Magee." In *Existentialists and Mystics: Writings on Philosophy and Literature*, 3–30. New York: Allen Lane, Penguin Press, 1998.

– "Metaphysics and Ethics." In *Existentialists and Mystics: Writings on Philosophy and Literature*, 59–75. New York: Penguin Press, 1998.

Nabokov, Vladimir. *Speak, Memory: An Autobiography Revisited*. New York: Vintage, 1989.

Neumann, Frederick. "Über das Lachen." In *Über das Lachen und Studien über den platonischen Sokrates*, 9–37. Den Haag: Martinus Nijhoff, 1971.

Nicolson, Harold. "The English Sense of Humour." In *The English Sense of Humour and other Essays*, 3–59. London: Constable and Company Limited, 1956.

Nowotny, Helga. "Dare to Know, Dare to Tell, Dare to Play," *Approaching Religion* 1, 2 (2011): 49–53.

– *An Orderly Mess*. New York: Central European University Press, 2017.

Nussbaum, Martha C. "Human Functioning and Social Justice: In Defense of Aristotelian Essentialism." *Political Theory* 20 (1992): 202–46.

– "Sex in the Head. Roger Scruton (1986). Sexual Desire: A Moral Philosophy of the Erotic." In *Philosophical Interventions: Reviews 1986–2011*, 27–35. New York: Oxford University Press, 2012.

Ortega y Gasset, José. "Tierras del Porvenir." In *Obras Completas. Tomo III (1917–1928)*. 6th ed., 481–5. Madrid: Revista de Occidente, 1966.

Orwell, George. *The Road to Wigan Pier*. London: Penguin Books, 2001.

Péguy, Charles. *Nous sommes tous à la frontière. Textes choisis par Hans Urs von Balthasar*. Einsiedeln: Johannes Verlag, 2014.

Pessoa, Fernando, "Three Prose Fragments." In *The Selected Prose of Fernando Pessoa*, edited and translated by Richard Zenith, 11–13. New York: Grove Press, 2001.

Plessner, Helmuth. "Zur Anthropologie der Musik." In *Ausdruck und menschliche Natur. Gesammelte Schriften VII*, 184–201. Frankfurt am Main: Suhrkamp Verlag, 1982.

– *Grenzen der Gemeinschaft. Eine Kritik des sozialen Radikalism. Gesammelte Schriften V*, 7–134. Frankfurt am Main: Suhrkamp Verlag, 1981.

– "On Human Expression." In *Phenomenological Psychology: The Dutch School*, edited by Joseph J. Kockelmans, 47–54. Dordrecht: Martinus Nijhoff, 1987.

– "Das Lächeln." In *Ausdruck und menschliche Natur. Gesammelte Schriften VII*, 421–33. Frankfurt am Main: Suhrkamp Verlag, 1982.

– *Laughing and Crying: A Study of the Limits of Human Behavior*. Translated by James Spencer Churchill and Marjorie Grene. Evanston: Northwestern University Press, 1970.

Plügge, Herbert. "Über die Arten der menschlichen Befangenheit." *Jahrbuch für Psychologie, Psychotherapie und Medizinische Anthropologie* 15 (1967): 1–12.

Postman, Neil. "Amusing Ourselves to Death." *etc: A Review of General Semantics* 42, 1 (spring 1985): 13–18.

– *Amusing Ourselves to Death: Public Discourse in the Age of Show Business*. London: Penguin, 2005.

Portmann, Adolf. "Spiel und Leben." In *Entlässt die Natur die Menschen. Gesammelte Ausätze zur Biologie und Anthropologie*, 230–52. Munich: R. Piper & Co. Verlag, 1971.

– "What Does the Living Form Mean to Us?" In *Essays in Philosophical Zoology by Adolf Portmann: The Living Form and the Seeing Eye*, translated by Richard B. Carter, 147–59. Lewiston, New York: Edwin Mellen Press, 1990.

Radermacher, Ludwig. *Weinen und Lachen. Studien über antikes Lebensgefühl*. Vienna: Rudolf M. Rohrer Verlag, 1947.

Rahner, Hugo. *Man at Play*. Translated by Brian Battershaw and Edward Quinn. Providence, Rhode Island: Cluny Media, 2019.

Reiners, Ludwig. *Stilkunst. Ein Lehrbuch Deutscher Prosa*. Munich: Verlag C.H. Beck, 2004.

Rensi, Giuseppe. *Contre le travail. Essai sur l'activité la plus honnie de l'homme*. Translated by Marie-José Tramuta. Paris: Allia, 2017.

– *Lettres spirituelles d'un philosophe sceptique*. Translated by Marie-José Tramuta. Paris: Allia, 2015.

Riezler, Kurt. "Play and Seriousness." *The Journal of Philosophy* 37 (1941): 505–17.

Ritter, Joachim. "Über das Lachen." In *Subjektivität*, 62–92. Frankfurt am Main: Suhrkamp Verlag, 1974.

Roditi, Georges. *L'esprit de perfection*. 13th. ed. Paris: Stock, 1996.

Rombach, Heinrich. *Strukturanthropologie. "Der menschliche Mensch."* Freiburg: Verlag Karl Alber, 1987.

Rothacker, Erich. *Geschichtsphilosophie*. Darmstadt: Wissenschaftliche Buchgesellschaft, 1971.

Rouet, Pascale. *André Isoir: Story of a Passionate Organist*. Le Vallier: Éditions Delatour France, 2020.

Rubik, Ernő. *Cubed: The Puzzle of Us All*. New York: Flatiron Book, 2020.

Ruch, Willibald. "Components of the Sense of Humor." In *Encyclopedia of Humor Studies*, edited by Salvatore Attardo, 680–2. Los Angeles: Sage Publications, 2014.

Rümke, H.C. "Divagations sur le problème: 'se fermer et s'ouvrir.'" In *Rencontre, Encounter, Begegnung. Contributions à une psychologie humaine dédiées au professeur F.J.J. Buytendijk*, 426–37. Utrecht: Uitgeverij Het Spectrum, 1957.

Saint-Exupéry, Antoine de. *Terre des hommes*. In *Œuvres complètes* I, 137–261. Paris: Gallimard, Bibliothèque de la Pléiade, 1994.

Saito, Yuriko. *Everyday Aesthetics*. Oxford: Oxford University Press, 2007.

Sansot, Pierre. *Du bon usage de la lenteur*. Paris: Payot & Rivages, 1998.

Santayana, George. *The Sense of Beauty: Being the Outline of Aesthetic Theory*. New York: Dover Publications, Inc., 1955.

Sartre, Jean-Paul. *L'être et le néant. Essai d'ontologie phénoménologique*. Paris: Gallimard, 1943.

Scheler, Max. *On the Eternal in Man*. Translated by Bernard Noble. New York: Harper & Brothers, 1960.

– "Phenomenology and the Theory of Cognition." In *Selected Philosophical Essays*, translated by David R. Lachterman, 136–201. Evanston: Northwestern University Press, 1973.

– "Shame and Feelings of Modesty." In *Person and Self-Value: Three Essays*, edited and translated by M.S. Frings, 1–85. Dordrecht: Martinus Nijhoff, 1987.

Schmitz, Kenneth L. "Sport and Play: Suspension of the Ordinary." In *Sport and the Body: A Philosophical Symposium*, edited by Ellen W. Gerber, 25–32. Philadelphia: Lea & Febiger, 1972.

Scruton, Roger. *Beauty: A Very Short Introduction*. Oxford: Oxford University Press, 2011.

– *Culture Counts: Faith and Feeling in a World Besieged*. New York: Encounter Books, 2007.

– *I Drink Therefore I Am: A Philosopher's Guide to Wine*. London: Bloomsbury Continuum, 2009.

– "Wine and Philosophy." *Decanter* (24 February, 2010): 57–9.

Seashore, Carl. E. "The Play Impulse and Attitude in Religion." *American Journal of Theology* 14 (1910): 505–20.

Serres, Michel. *Morales espiègles*. Paris: Éditions Le Pommier – Humensis, 2019.

– *Le Tiers-Instruit*. Paris: Gallimard, 1992.

Shils, Edward. "The Virtue of Civility." In *The Virtue of Civility: Selected Essays on Liberalism, Tradition, and Civil Society*, edited by Steven Grosby, 320–55. Indianapolis: Liberty Fund, 1997.

Sicart, Miguel. *Play Matters*. Cambridge: MIT PRESS, 2014.

Simmel, Georg. "Flirtation." In *On Women, Sexuality, and Love*, translated by Guy Oakes, 133–52. New Haven: Yale University Press, 1984.

Spaemann, Robert. *Basic Moral Concepts*. Translated by T.J. Armstrong. London: Routledge, 1991.

Stevenson, Charles L. "The Nature of Ethical Disagreement." In *Facts and Values*, 1–9. New Haven: Yale University Press, 1963.

Stevenson, Robert Louis. "Child's Play." In *Virginibus Puerisque and Other Papers*, 127–39. Harmondsworth: Penguin Books, 1946.

Straus, Erwin W. "The Forms of Spatiality." In *Phenomenological Psychology* (1966). Reprint ed., translated by Erling Eng, 3–37. New York: Garland, 1980.

– "The Miser." In *Patterns of the Life-World*, edited by James M. Edie, Francis H. Parker, and Calvin O. Schrag, 157–79. Evanston: Northwestern University Press, 1970.

– "The Pathology of Compulsion." In *Phenomenological Psychology* (1966). Reprint ed., translated by Erling Eng, 296–329. New York: Garland, 1980.

– *The Primary World of Senses: A Vindication of Sensory Experience*. Translated by Jacob Needleman. New York: Free Press of Glencoe, 1963.

Tellenbach, Hubertus. "Am Leitfaden des Leibes zu einer anthropologischen Physiologie." *Jahrbuch für Psychologie, Psychotherapie und Medizinische Anthropologie* 18 (1970): 16–20.

– "La réalité, le comique et l'humour." In *La réalité, le comique et l'humour, suivi des actes du colloque réunis par Yves Pelicier: Autour de la pensée de Tellenbach*, translated by Philippe Forget, 7–18. Paris: Economica, 1981.

Thomas Aquinas. *Commentary on Aristotle's* De Anima. Translated by Robert Pasnau, New Haven: Yale University Press, 1999.

Thomas, Lewis. "Humanities and Science." In *Late Night Thoughts on Listening to Mahler's Ninth Symphony*, 143–55. New York: Viking Press, 184.

Tolstoy, Leo. *War and Peace*. Translated by Constance Garnett. New York: Book-of-the-Month Club, 1985.

Ulrich, Ferdinand. *Der Mensch als Anfang. Zur philosophischen Anthropologie der Kindheit*. Einsiedeln: Johannes Verlag, 1970.

Ungar, Michael. *Too Safe for Their Own Good: How Risk and Responsibility Help Teens Thrive*. Toronto: McClelland & Stewart, 2007.

Valéry, Paul. "Mélange." In *Œuvres I*, 285–339. Paris: Gallimard, Bibliothèque de la Pléiade, 1957.

Van Doren, Mark. "Joseph and His Brothers: A Comedy in Four Parts." In *The Happy Critic and Other Essays*, 71–87. Edinburgh and London: Oliver & Boyd, 1961.

Waugh, Evelyn. "Travel – and Escape from Your Friends." In *The Essays, Articles and Reviews of Evelyn Waugh*, edited by Donat Gallagher, 133–4. Boston: Little, Brown and Company, 1984.

Weil, Simone. *The Need for Roots: Prelude to a Declaration of Duties towards Mankind*. Translated by A.F. Wills. London: Ark Paperbacks, 1987.

Weiss, Gabriele. "Sich verausgabende Spieler und andere vereinnahmende Falschspieler. Das Spiel zwischen Möglichkeit und Wirklichkeit in ästhetischen Lebensformen." In Alfred Schäfer and Christine Thomson, eds., *Spiel*, 35–61. Paderborn: Ferdinand Schöningh, 2014.

Welte, Bernhard. "Dasein im Symbol des Spiels." In *Zwischen Zeit und Ewigkeit. Abhandlungen und Versuche*, 96–108. Freiburg: Herder Verlag, 1982.

Whitehead, Alfred North. *Science and the Modern World*. Harmondsworth: Penguin Books, 1938.

Winnicott, D.W. *Playing and Reality*. London: Penguin Book, 1974.

Wittgenstein, Ludwig. *Culture and Value*. Edited by G.H. von Wright in collaboration with Heikki Nyman. Chicago: University of Chicago Press, 1984.

Worsley, F.A. *Shackleton's Boat Journey*. Edinburgh: Birlinn Limited, 2007.

Zutt, Jürg. "Die innere Haltung." In *Auf dem Wege zu einer anthropologischen Psychiatrie. Gesammelte Aufsätze*, 1–88. Berlin: Springer-Verlag, 1963.

Zweig, Stefan. *Twenty-Four Hours in the Life of a Woman*. Translated by Anthea Bell. London: Pushkin Press, 2011.

Index

abstractness, 6, 89; abstract person, 114

adaptation, 68, 71; reciprocal initiative and, 44

addiction, 35–6, 53

adventure: body's potential for, 57; science as, 66

aesthetic: awareness nurtures playfulness, 137; encounter while making something, 138–9; enjoyment, 134–5; experience while using objects, 137–8; relation to objects, 135–6; responsiveness, 134–40; skill and practical purpose, 139

Alain (Émile-Auguste Chartier), 33, 75, 125

Al-Sabouni, Marwa, 160n27

amateur, 122–3; musicians, 62; praise of, 123, 159n30

animated realities, 44–5, 110, 143; emotional relation to, 50–1

anthropology: of childhood, 141; of everyday life, 93–4; philosophical, 14

Arendt, Hannah, 63

Arnheim, Rudolf, 66, 128

art of living, 123–6

atmosphere, 32, 37, 40, 46, 136–7; attitude as an overall, 32; of the city, 115–16; of collaboration, 66; of common understanding and conviviality, 100; created by humour and music, 146; created by a song, 112; created by a teacher, 66; of ease and gaiety, 28; of excitement, 53; forbidding, 6; of inner peacefulness, 133; oppressive, 5–6; personal, 18–19; of seriousness, 40; stimulating, 66–7; synchrony with, 113; of trust, 65–6; of usefulness, 107–8

attitude: adopted instantaneously, 22; adopted voluntarily, 15; behind teaching, 66; bodily, 16–19; constitution of the, 23–4; defines human relations, 24–5; as an enduring disposition, 15, 18, 25; in everyday life, 4; foundational, 23; growing into, 20–1; as a guiding *ethos*, 24, 32; toward human life, 4; inner, 18–19, 21; as the mirror of the person, 19; national, 22; of non-attachment, 68; observable, 18; phenomenological, 15; as the quality of a presence, 18; as a response, 25–6; serene, 71; social, 20–1; undergoes transformation, 22–3; unexpected, 25; unworried, 71

attitude of play: absence of, 5–7; allows us to see, 38–9; of the amateur, 122–3; and the art of living, 126; being immune to, 5, 7–8, 10; characteristics, 28–9; dispels tension, 56; educational